Strategies to Reduce Hospital Mortality in Lower and Middle Income Countries (LMICs) and Resource-Limited Settings

Edited by Jasneth Mullings,
Camille-Ann Thoms-Rodriguez,
Affette M. McCaw-Binns and Tomlin Paul

Published in London, United Kingdom

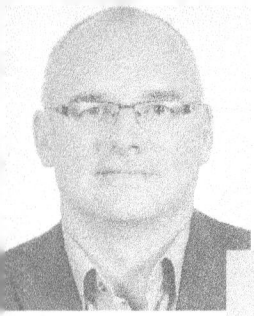
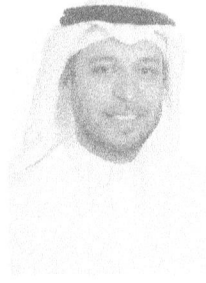
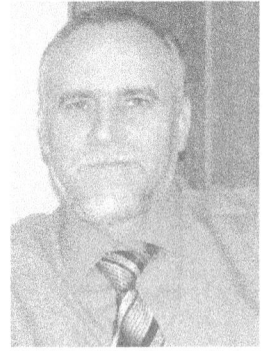
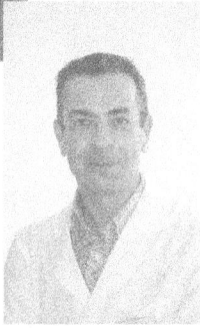
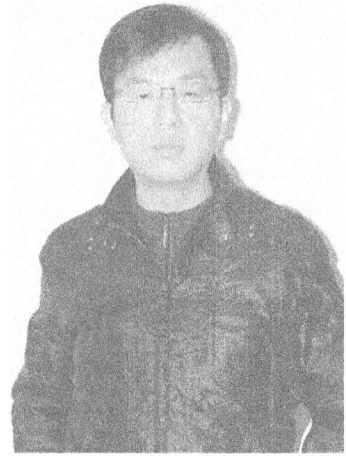
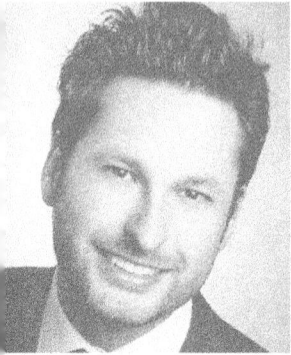
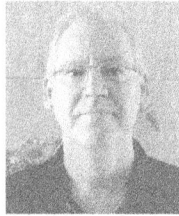

IntechOpen

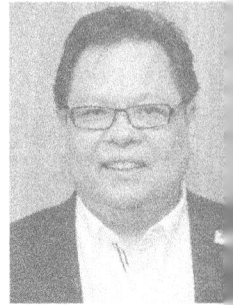
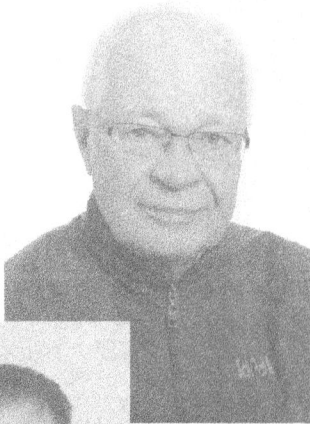
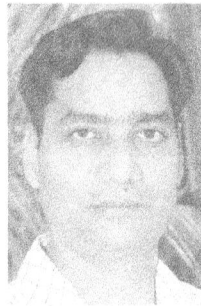
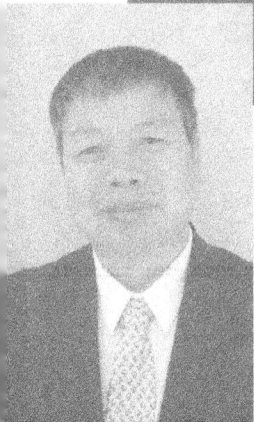
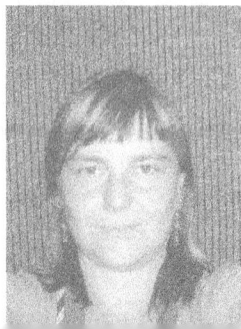
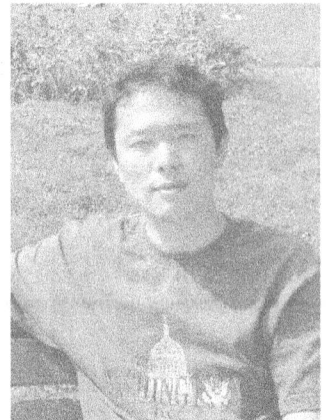

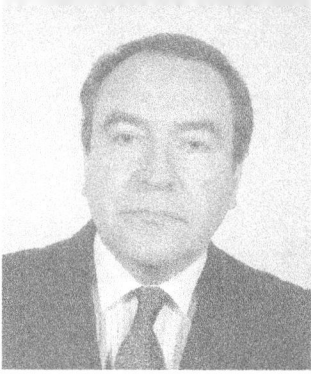

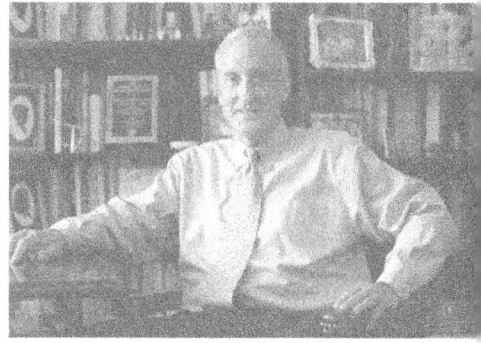

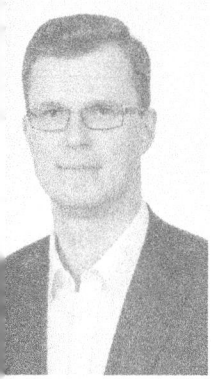

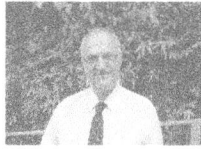

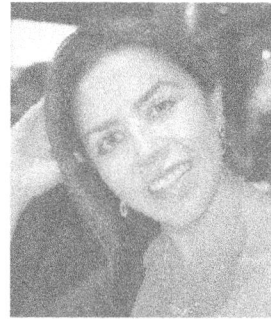

Supporting open minds since 2005

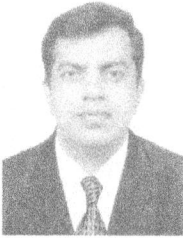

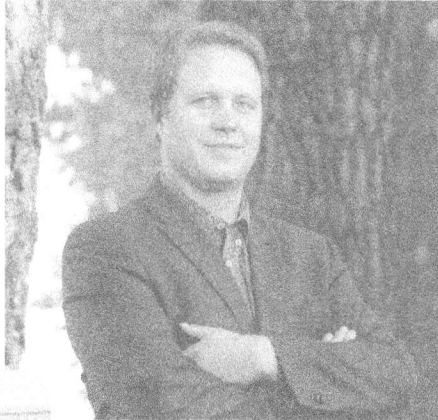

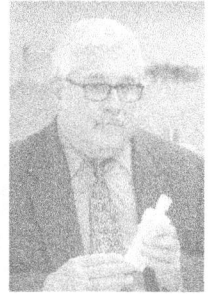

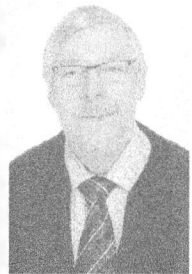

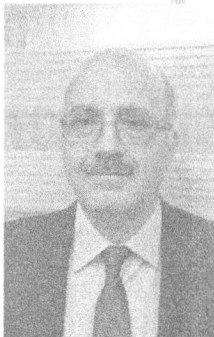

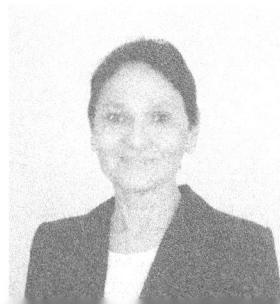

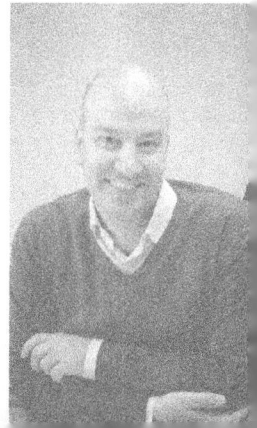

Strategies to Reduce Hospital Mortality in Lower and Middle Income Countries (LMICs) and Resource-Limited Settings
http://dx.doi.org/10.5772/intechopen.73957
Edited by Jasneth Mullings, Camille-Ann Thoms-Rodriguez, Affette M. McCaw-Binns and Tomlin Paul

Assistant to the Editort(s): Antoinette Barton-Gooden

Contributors
Martin Lankoandé, Papougnezambo Bonkoungou, Souleymane Oubian, Ghislain Somda, Joachim Sanou, Jasneth Mullings, Donnette Wright, Monique Lynch, Geovanni Franklin, Joseph Plummer, Mark Newnham, Timothy Henry

Notice
Statements and opinions expressed in the chapters are these of the individual contributors and not necessarily those of the editors or publisher. No responsibility is accepted for the accuracy of information contained in the published chapters. The publisher assumes no responsibility for any damage or injury to persons or property arising out of the use of any materials, instructions, methods or ideas contained in the book.

First published in London, United Kingdom, 2019 by IntechOpen
IntechOpen is the global imprint of INTECHOPEN LIMITED, registered in England and Wales, registration number: 11086078, The Shard, 25th floor, 32 London Bridge Street
London, SE19SG – United Kingdom
Printed in Croatia

British Library Cataloguing-in-Publication Data
A catalogue record for this book is available from the British Library

Additional hard and PDF copies can be obtained from orders@intechopen.com

Strategies to Reduce Hospital Mortality in Lower and Middle Income Countries (LMICs) and Resource-Limited Settings
Edited by Jasneth Mullings, Camille-Ann Thoms-Rodriguez, Affette M. McCaw-Binns and Tomlin Paul
p. cm.
Print ISBN 978-1-83880-933-1
Online ISBN 978-1-83962-225-0
eBook (PDF) ISBN 978-1-83962-226-7

We are IntechOpen,
the world's leading publisher of
Open Access books
Built by scientists, for scientists

4,300+
Open access books available

116,000+
International authors and editors

130M+
Downloads

Our authors are among the

151
Countries delivered to

Top 1%
most cited scientists

12.2%
Contributors from top 500 universities

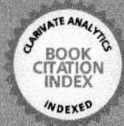

Interested in publishing with us?
Contact book.department@intechopen.com

Numbers displayed above are based on latest data collected.
For more information visit www.intechopen.com

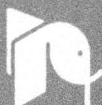

Meet the editors

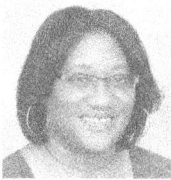

Dr. Jasneth Mullings is a researcher/scientist/lecturer in the Faculty of Medical Sciences, The University of the West Indies (UWI), Mona, Jamaica. Based in the Health Research Resource Unit, Dr. Mullings provides research support to faculty and graduate students. She has a master's degree in Public Health/Health Education and was the first PhD Epidemiology graduate of UWI (2013). She has received academic awards for her work. Her current research interests are mental health, urban health, community health, and related interventions. Her publication record includes one book, two book chapters, 10 journal articles, 27 abstracts, and 12 technical reports. She has held membership in the International Society for Urban Health and International Society for Environmental Epidemiology.

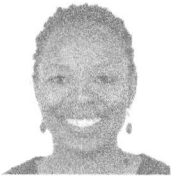

Dr. Thoms-Rodriguez has a MD in Microbiology. She lectures at the University of the West Indies, Mona, Jamaica, specializing in Medical Microbiology with special interest in infectious diseases, antibiotic resistance, and control of healthcare-associated infections. She has pursued specialist training in infectious diseases, infection control, and epidemiology surveillance. Dr. Thoms-Rodriguez has published articles in peer-reviewed, refereed journals and has made numerous presentations at international conferences. She recently co-authored a book chapter, "Bacterial Infections in the Oral Cavity: Characterization, Diagnosis, Treatment and Prevention" in *Clinical Microbiology for the General Dentist*. She holds membership in several learned societies and associations, including the American Society for Microbiology and International Society Infectious Diseases, and is currently President of the Caribbean Association of Clinical Microbiologists.

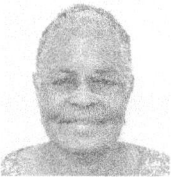

Dr. McCaw-Binns (BA [NYU], MPH [Tulane], PhD [Bristol]) is Professor of Reproductive Health and Epidemiology in the Department of Community Health and Psychiatry, University of the West Indies, Mona, Jamaica. Her maternal and perinatal health research has generated more than 100 peer-reviewed publications, informing the development of maternal mortality surveillance, clinical guidelines and health promotion tools for pre-eclampsia, and establishment of high-risk antenatal clinics and other services aimed at ending preventable maternal and perinatal deaths in Jamaica. Her global service includes collaborations with the Pan American Health Organization (PAHO), United Nations Population Fund (UNFPA), and UN women, among others. Since 2006 she has assisted the WHO Special Programme of Research, Development and Research Training in Human Reproduction to improve measurement, surveillance, and strategies to enhance global maternal health and survival.

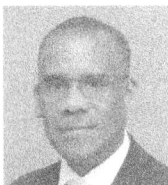

Dr. Tomlin Paul is Dean of the Faculty of Medical Sciences, University of the West Indies (UWI), Mona, Jamaica. He has MB, BS, and MPH degrees and is a Diplomate of the Faculty of Public Health Medicine, Royal College of Physicians. His research interests include medical education and social accountability. He is a fellow of the Academy of Medical Educators, UK, and has served as a consultant to the Pan American Health Organization and medical schools in the region. He has worked in the primary care setting in Jamaica and is an advocate for quality improvement in health and education systems.

Contents

Preface

In 2019, the World Health Organization (WHO) named the following top ten threats to global health: air pollution and climate change, non-communicable diseases, global influenza pandemic, fragile and vulnerable settings, antimicrobial resistance, Ebola and other high-threat pathogens, weak primary health care, vaccine hesitancy, dengue, and HIV. In 2017, approximately 56 million deaths were recorded worldwide. Many of the deaths from these conditions and exposures on the WHO's watch list occur in hospitals.

This book examines the issue of hospital mortality from the perspective of Low- and Middle-Income Countries (LMICs) and presents a mix of strategies in support of strengthening health systems and reducing mortality. The strategies for reducing hospital mortality are shown in this book to lie within a clinical-public health nexus and, as such, are not only the domain of the hospitalist or clinical administrator. Quality of care is an important overarching theme within which a sound argument on hospital mortality reduction can be built. Achieving such quality of care calls for consideration of a structured system for quality management supported by appropriate epidemiological and management information.

This book targets academics, clinicians, health administrators, and policy makers, as well as students of public health. It engages these groups in an examination of health conditions, clinical management tools, and other related issues that require policy and programmatic interventions best suited to the population health realm.

The WHO (2011) defined health literacy as the degree to which individuals have the capacity to obtain, process, and understand basic health information and services needed to make basic health decisions for themselves and their loved ones. Health literacy and its relationship with health outcomes is well placed in the discussion of hospital mortality and appropriate interventions for researchers and healthcare professionals to reduce the negative impact on these outcomes. There is need for research to advance the conceptualization of health literacy in reducing hospital mortality and morbidity.

The discussion around surgical care and applying guidelines and protocols in patient care is much needed for LMICs. It is relevant to overall hospital mortality reduction as such interventions around standardizing care are needed and will bring similar returns in all areas of a hospital where high-volume, complex care takes place. The surgical environment has become more complex with a wider range of procedures and changes in approaches and use of technology. Additionally, patient expectations have grown. This is more important in developing countries where access to resources are limited but access to information globally has improved. There is no doubt that the streamlining of the patient:-treatment:-outcome continuum can be made better with the use of various standard operating procedures, such as the use of guidelines, protocols, and checklists with a multidisciplinary team where all stakeholders are actively engaged.

The importance of nutrition across the lifespan is well recognized. Clinical management approaches and algorithms for nutritional management procedures in the hospital setting are discussed in the book. However, resource-limited environments pose a threat to implementing well-known nutritional adequacy interventions that can reduce hospital mortality.

With the changing epidemiological profile and a growing elderly population, there is a need to examine the health system's response to the older population. A special area to be highlighted is the causes and prognosis of older patients admitted in ICU. Despite the severity of many of the conditions contributing to mortality, there is a need for application of quality management protocols in this setting.

Currently, three out of four people die from a chronic non-communicable disease (CNCD), and 40% are premature deaths occurring between ages 30 years and 69 years. In considering mortality as a key indicator of the health of a population, with life expectancy a commonly reported measure, it is noted that there are significant regional differences in global life expectancy at birth. LMICs need to have evidence-based models that are relevant to their setting and aimed at reducing the associated morbidity burden and mortality in these resource-limited environments. Policy development around critical issues in these countries is an important step to reducing mortality across the demographic spectrum. From a quality perspective, there is likely to be an overall positive effect of a robust hospital quality-of-care system in LMICs.

On behalf of the editorial team, I wish to thank the authors who made their contribution to this work and trust that this publication will help to open up this conversation across the academic-public discourse nexus. If this publication can support action to reduce hospital mortality, increase healthy life expectancy, and improve quality of life in resource-limited settings across the globe, the contributions of the authors and editors would have given added value and meaning to this effort.

Dr. Jasneth Mullings
The University of the West Indies,
Mona, Kingston, Jamaica

Section 1

Reducing Hospital Mortality: Programmatic and Policy Interventions

Chapter 1

Introductory Chapter: Mortality and Quality of Care Systems in LMICs

Jasneth Mullings, Affette McCaw Binns,
Camille-Ann Thoms-Rodriguez,
Antoinette Barton-Gooden and Tomlin Paul

1. Mortality and risk factors: the global picture

Mortality data is a key indicator of the health of a population, with life expectancy being a commonly reported measure. Most recent estimates (2015) place global life expectancy at birth at 71.4 years but with significant regional differences. Improvements in life expectancy over the last few decades are reflected in the 55% of global deaths which occurred among older persons 65 years and over (moving from 41% in 1990). This development is a marker of socioeconomic development and progress in the reduction of premature deaths [1].

In 2017 approximately 56 million deaths were recorded and of that number non-communicable diseases (NCDs); communicable, maternal, neonatal and nutritional diseases; and injuries accounted for 72.3, 19.3, and 4.6% of deaths, respectively [2]. Cause-specific mortality for the top 10 leading causes of death was attributed to cardiovascular diseases (32.26%), cancers (16.32%), respiratory diseases (6.48%), diabetes (5.83%), dementia (4.36%), lower respiratory infections (4.35%), neonatal deaths (3.16%), diarrheal diseases (3.03%), road incidents (2.45%), and liver disease (2.3%) [2].

Globally, the predominant risk factors for mortality are preventable and include high blood pressure, smoking, high blood sugar, high body mass index (obesity), high cholesterol, outdoor air pollution, alcohol use, household air pollution, low fruit diets, and low vegetable diet. While both men and women have metabolic and behavioral risk factors for early death and disability, the leading behavioral risk factors for men were smoking and alcohol consumption, while for women metabolic risk factors were predominant (e.g., high systolic blood pressure, glucose, and body mass index) [2]. The association between nutrition and NCDs may have arguably originated in utero [3], and an increased awareness of epigenetics has thickened the discussion around NCDs and associated mortality. Discussions on health disparities and NCDs have also become increasingly relevant, especially given global economic disparities and social risks which directly impact on the poor, marginalized and other vulnerable populations. This is oftentimes compounded by deficiencies in health literacy and inadequate integration of evidence-based models in health care.

While non-communicable diseases have largely accounted for global deaths, acute and chronic respiratory conditions remain the major threats to survival. In 2016, the top two leading causes of death in low-income countries were non-communicable diseases—lower respiratory infections and diarrhoeal diseases [2].

Among the many respiratory conditions that contribute to hospital mortality, infectious causes are reported to account for the largest proportion [4]. The Global Burden of Diseases, Injuries, and Risk Factors (GBD) Study (2015) reported in the Lancet Infectious Diseases (2017) that, worldwide, the fifth cause of death overall was attributable to lower respiratory tract infections [4]. Over 50% of these deaths (totaling 1,517,388) in all ages were attributable to pneumococcal pneumonia. The impact of this was disproportionately seen among various age groups with the greatest impact in childhood [4]. Vaccination, proper nutrition and a reduction in exposure to contaminated air were important strategies that resulted in a reduction in mortality in children [3]. Other important infectious agents associated with significant morbidity and mortality include *Haemophilus influenzae* serotype B, *Mycobacterium tuberculosis* complex (MTBc), influenza virus, and the respiratory syncytial virus with MTBc infections being among the top 10 causes of death globally [5]. Tuberculosis has had a resurgence in recent times, associated with the HIV/AIDS epidemic. Management of these conditions has been further complicated by the development of multidrug-resistant strains which further contribute to significant morbidity and mortality [5].

2. Health disparities and the growing burden in LMICs

Health disparities between high- and low-income countries are reflected in the leading causes of death in low-income countries being communicable, maternal, neonatal, and nutritional diseases compared to non-communicable diseases (e.g., ischemic heart disease, stroke, and lung cancer) in high-income countries. Lower-middle, upper-middle and high-income countries all reported ischemic heart disease and stroke as the top two leading causes of death. Notably, however, ischemic heart disease was the third leading cause of death in low-income countries, signaling an epidemiological transition [6] (**Table 1**).

The prevalence of chronic non-communicable diseases (CNCD) in lower middle-income countries (LMICs) is burdensome. Currently, three out of four people die from a CNCD, and 40% are premature, occurring between 30 and 69 years [7]. The drivers of these diseases are well documented and include both behavioral and biological factors, which are challenging to address when compounded with needed health system strengthening. Notwithstanding, the latter may be easier to address strategically through policy implementation, while the former will need an ecological approach that addresses cultural and economic nuances that are inherent in LMICs.

The economic fallout from the global NCD burden over the next 20 years is estimated at a cumulative loss output of US$ 47 trillion, representing a value of 75% of global gross domestic product at 2010. The forces of population growth and ageing are expected to increase the number of persons affected by NCDs, thereby increasing healthcare costs and reducing productivity globally. Cardiovascular disease and mental health conditions are the major contributors to the economic burden. The largest share of the burden will be borne by high-income countries. However, the scale of the impact in developing countries will increase as a result of population growth and economic challenges [8]. LMICs are increasingly being challenged by the lack of resources and inadequate infrastructure and health systems to effectively respond to the NCD epidemic, while many are simultaneously battling emerging and re-emerging communicable diseases. Jamaica and Burkina Faso are among two of the countries classified as LMICs, albeit at different ends of the spectrum, but facing grave economic and social challenges. Experiences from both countries are shared in this book.

Rank	High-income countries	Upper-middle income countries	Lower-middle income countries	Low-income countries
1	Ischemic heart disease	Ischemic heart disease	Ischemic heart disease	Lower respiratory infections
2	Stroke	Stroke	Stroke	Diarrhoeal diseases
3	Alzheimer disease and other dementias	Chronic obstructive pulmonary disease	Lower respiratory infections	Ischemic heart disease
4	Trachea, bronchus, and lung cancers	Trachea, bronchus, lung cancers	Chronic obstructive pulmonary disease	HIV/AIDS
5	Chronic obstructive pulmonary disease	Alzheimer disease and other dementias	Tuberculosis	Stroke
6	Lower respiratory infections	Lower respiratory infections	Diarrhoeal diseases	Malaria
7	Colon and rectum cancers	Diabetes mellitus	Diabetes mellitus	Tuberculosis
8	Diabetes mellitus	Road injury	Pre-term birth complications	Pre-term birth complications
9	Kidney disease	Liver cancer	Cirrhosis of the liver	Birth asphyxia and birth trauma
10	Breast cancer	Stomach cancer	Road injury	Road injury

Source: World Health Organization [6].

Table 1.
Top ten causes of death by income group, 2016.

Burkina Faso in Africa has a population of 18,450,000 and life expectancy at birth of 60 years. Communicable diseases account for 5 of the top 10 causes of death, the top 3 of which are lower respiratory infections (14%), malaria (10%) and diarrheal disease (6%) [9]. These data reflect a country in what Omran described as the second stage of the epidemiological transition—'Age of Receding Pandemics' [10]—characterized by a shift from primarily infectious diseases to include non-communicable diseases such as stroke (6%), ischemic heart disease (4%), and road injury (3%) [9]. Burkina Faso is classified as a low-income country by the World Bank, with an economy which is heavily reliant on agriculture and vulnerable to external shocks and internal political instability. Ranked 144 out of 157 countries on the new World Bank Human Capital Index, Burkina Faso is severely challenged by the impact of the twin epidemics of communicable and non-communicable diseases [11].

Home to 2.9 million persons, Jamaica, the largest island in the English-speaking Caribbean, has a life expectancy at birth of 76 years and is classified as an upper middle-income economy. In spite of this, the country has struggled with low growth, high public debt and vulnerability to external shocks from global economic forces and natural disasters such as floods and hurricanes [12]. Across the Caribbean, governments are paying increased attention to the impact of NCDs on sustainable development. In the case of Jamaica, GDP output loss due to the four leading NCDs (cardiovascular disease, cancer, chronic respiratory disease, and diabetes) and mental health conditions is projected at US$ 18.45 billion over the 2015–2030 period. As a singular factor, cardiovascular disease is expected to account for 20% of this loss [13]. Furthermore, NCDs and mental health conditions are projected to reduce annual GDP by 3.9% between 2015 and 2030. Regional government commitment to policy and programs to address the NCD epidemic is relatively strong but challenged by economic realities.

3. Hospital mortality data systems: measuring quality of care

As the world faces a multiplicity of health challenges, the World Health Organization is following its 2019 watch list of 10 threats to global health: air pollution and climate change, non-communicable diseases, global influenza pandemic, fragile and vulnerable settings, antimicrobial resistance, Ebola and other high-threat pathogens, weak primary health care, vaccine hesitancy, dengue, and HIV [14].

Many of the deaths from these conditions and exposures occur in hospitals. Hospital mortality data is an important source of information to support health system strengthening globally by enabling monitoring and improvements in quality of care [15]. Robust public health planning requires the availability of timely and accurate data on the leading causes of death and disability.

The World Health Organization reports that cause-of-death statistics from hospital sources and other sources form the basis of statistics on the health of a population. This information is used for development planning by governments, researchers, and donor agencies and is often used to track progress on national and international development goals. However, the issue of accuracy has remained a concern in many jurisdictions. Addressing this issue requires an expanded awareness of the public health value of correct certification and coding of hospital deaths and the proper maintenance of hospital records to facilitate improved diagnoses and treatment. Continuous monitoring and evaluation of cause-of-death certification and coding and medical record practices is also necessary to support useful and effective national mortality data systems [16, 17].

Given the challenges in data quality and utilization for hospital performance metrics, experts recommend the following to improve the quality and use of hospital mortality data:

- Regular national audits of mortality with feedback to hospitals to address gaps in reporting and analysis

- Training programs for doctors and medical students on cause-of-death certification and coding

- Alignment of hospital cause-specific mortality reporting with disease surveillance and response programs

- Strengthening of maternal and perinatal death surveillance and response, focusing on lessons learned to improve quality and safety

- Capacity building for clinical and population health epidemiology to enable improved sophistication in analyses [18, 19].

4. Strategies, guidelines and lessons for LMICs

Persons requiring hospital admission are those whose illnesses require professional supervision. The book outlines strategies to enable the best possible outcome with interventions focused on improving the health literacy of the patients and ensuring that their nutrition is optimal, ranging from the very preterm infant to end-of-life care for the elderly.

An informed consumer improves the likelihood of developing a cooperative relationship between the general public and the health team. Lynch and Franklin discuss health literacy, or the capacity of the patient to obtain, process and understand basic health information and services needed to make the basic health decisions for themselves and their loved ones. They outline what the concept of health literacy means, especially its limited prevalence, and explore possible strategies to improve its contribution to reducing hospital mortality and morbidity.

Global evidence suggest that efforts to standardize care for all patients help to improve outcomes, and as such there is a growing support for the development of clinical guidelines, which are adapted to local conditions, clear protocols for care and the use of checklists to ensure that the care process is consistent. With increasing life expectancy, few patients present with a single health problem nor is addressing even a specific problem the singular responsibility of one professional, so the building of multidisciplinary teams and improving the facility with which members of the health team work together for the good of the patient are discussed by Plummer and colleagues.

Supportive care while in hospital requires attention to optimize the contribution of adequate nutrition to the patient's recovery and health maintenance going forward. Wright argues that this requires attention to the professional, skill, knowledge and experience of the health team as these are important correlates that may modify patient outcomes. Even in well-resourced settings, this aspect of care does not receive the attention it deserves; however the authors argue that in under-resourced developed states, it is important to capitalize on this valuable asset which can assist health teams to realize positive gains in patient survival through the establishment of good policies and standards for care.

Life-threatening complications require tertiary care, including access to intensive care services. Once these units are established, we need to understand the factors associated with adverse outcomes and ensure that strategies are put in place to address those preventable complications. Martin and colleagues explore the Burkina Faso experience and lessons to reduce mortality among the elderly.

Developing evidence-based models which are contextually relevant for LMICs is critical to reducing associated burden and mortality in these resource-limited environments.

Addressing hospital mortality is a complex task and the span of issues covered in this book shows that there is a bigger frame within which all strategies should be considered. As much as the hospital is an entity strongly focused on clinical care, it remains a part of the wider health system. The book chapters cut across issues of personal risk and resource considerations to environmental exposures and policies affecting education and health literacy. Placing the strategies collectively within a broad field frame begs the question of the role of the hospital as a socially accountable institution.

While the strategies could be seen as acting upon a situation occurring within the institution, the institution as a whole must be seen as having collective responsibility and scope for action. Overall, social accountability is an effective strategy for improving the quality and performance of health-care service providers and institutions and it has been shown to have better status in private hospitals compared to public and teaching ones [20]. In low- and middle-income countries, such as Jamaica, the majority of hospital care of the population is delivered through public hospitals. As such, efforts to improve the overall social accountability must be a priority overarching strategy for reducing mortality.

A big part of such strategic intervention on social accountability in hospitals will be tied to having adequate corporate governance and corporate strategy social responsibility [21]. Stakeholders' demands must be met and there must be a culture of performance, conformance, and responsibility. Hospitals, seeking to improve health outcomes in a cost-effective manner, should consider preventive measures in developing intervention strategies. This is an important consideration around the strategies discussed in this book. Placing the hospital in a role to also address social determinants [22] may seem a misfit with its core mission. However, if real gains are to be made in LMICs with limited resources and the threat of stagnation within the epidemiological transition, a socially accountable framework must be considered to bring synergies with the overall health system and much needed and added value to individual strategies.

The issues covered in the book create a framework from which policies may be developed to improve the prevention and management of disease, with the hope of reducing the associated hospital mortality.

Author details

Jasneth Mullings*, Affette McCaw Binns, Camille-Ann Thoms-Rodriguez, Antoinette Barton-Gooden and Tomlin Paul
The University of the West Indies, Mona, Jamaica

*Address all correspondence to: jasneth.mullings@uwimona.edu.jm

IntechOpen

References

[1] United Nations, Department
of Economic and Social Affairs,
Population Division. World Mortality
2017—Data Booklet (ST/ESA/
SER.A/412). 2017. Available from:
https://www.un.org/en/development/
desa/population/publications/pdf/
mortality/World-Mortality-2017-Data-
Booklet.pdf

[2] Institute of Health Metrics and
Evaluation (IHME). Global Burden
of Disease Study 2017. 2018. Available
from: http://www.healthdata.org/sites/
default/files/files/policy_report/2019/
GBD_2017_Booklet.pdf

[3] Baroukil R, Gluckman P, Grandjean P,
Hanson M, Heindel J. Developmental
origins of non-communicable disease:
Implications for research and public
health. Environmental Health.
2012;**11**:42

[4] GBD 2015 LRI Collaborators.
Estimates of the global, regional,
and national morbidity, mortality,
and aetiologies of lower respiratory
tract infections in 195 countries: A
systematic analysis for the Global
Burden of Disease Study 2015.
The Lancet Infectious Diseases.
2017;**17**(11):1133-1161. DOI: 10.1016/
S1473-3099(17)30396-1

[5] WHO Media Centre. Tuberculosis.
The World Health Organization
[Online]. 2018. Available from: https://
www.who.int/en/news-room/fact-
sheets/detail/tuberculosis# [Accessed:
September 18, 2018]

[6] World Health Organization. The
Top 10 Causes of Death. https://www.
who.int/news-room/fact-sheets/detail/
the-top-10-causes-of-death

[7] Luciani S. Non-communicable
diseases: Regional plan of action and
commitments to strengthening NCD
Management. In: PAHO Meeting:

Increasing Access to NCD Medicine in
the Caribbean; February 22-23, 2017

[8] Bloom D, Cafiero E, Jané-Llopis E,
Abrahams-Gessel S, Bloom L, Fathima S,
et al. The Global Economic Burden of
Noncommunicable Diseases. Geneva:
World Economic Forum; 2011

[9] Centers for Disease Control. CDC in
Burkina Faso. Available from: https://
www.cdc.gov/globalhealth/countries/
burkinafaso/pdf/BurkinaFaso_
Factsheet.pdf

[10] Omran AR. The epidemiologic
transition. The Milbank Memorial Fund
Quarterly. 1971;**49**:509-538

[11] World Bank. The World Bank in
Burkina Faso. Available from: http://
www.worldbank.org/en/country/
burkinafaso/overview

[12] World Bank. The World Bank in
Jamaica. Available from: http://www.
worldbank.org/en/country/jamaica/
overview

[13] Bloom DE, Chen S, McGovern ME.
The economic burden of
noncommunicable diseases and mental
health conditions: Results for Costa
Rica, Jamaica, and Peru. Revista
Panamericana de Salud Pública.
2018;**42**:e18. DOI: 10.26633/
RPSP.2018.18

[14] World Health Organization.
Ten Threats to Global Health in
2019. Available from: https://
www.who.int/emergencies/
ten-threats-to-global-health-in-2019

[15] Goodacre S, Campbell M,
Carter A. What do hospital mortality
rates tell us about quality of care?
Emergency Medicine Journal.
2015;**32**:244-247

[16] Rampatige R, Mikkelsen L,
Hernandez B, Riley I, Lopez A. Hospital

cause-of-death statistics: What should we make of them? Bulletin of the World Health Organization. 2014;**92**:3-3A. DOI: 10.2471/BLT.13.134106

[17] McCaw-Binns A, Holder Y, Mullings J. Certification of coroners cases by pathologists would improve the completeness of death registration in Jamaica. Journal of Clinical Epidemiology. 2015;**68**(9):979-987. DOI: 10.1016/j.jclinepi.2014.11.026. Epub: February 7, 2015

[18] English M, Mwaniki P, Julius T, Chepkirui M, Gathara D, Ouma P, et al. Hospital mortality—A neglected but rich source of information supporting the transition to higher quality health systems in low- and middle-income countries. BMC Medicine. 2018;**16**:32. DOI: 10.1186/s12916-018-1024-8. PMCID: PMC5833062. Published Online: March 1, 2018

[19] McCaw-Binns AM, Mullings JA, Holder Y. Vital registration and under-reporting of maternal mortality in Jamaica. International Journal of Gynecology & Obstetrics. 2015;**128**:62-67. DOI: 10.1016/j.ijgo.2014.07.023

[20] Mahmoudi G, Jahani MA, Rostami FH, Mahmoudjanloo S, Nikbakht H. Comparing the levels of hospital's social accountability: Based on ownership. International Journal of Healthcare Management. 2018;**11**(4):319-324. DOI: 10.1080/20479700.2017.1417074

[21] Brandão C, Rego G, Duarte I, Nunes R. Social responsibility: A new paradigm of hospital governance? Health Care Analysis. 2012;**21**(4):390-402. DOI: 10.1007/s10728-012-0206-3

[22] Sullivan HR. Hospitals' obligations to address social determinants of health. AMA Journal of Ethics. 2019;**21**(3):E248-E258. DOI: 10.1001/amajethics.2019.248

Chapter 2

Health Literacy: An Intervention to Improve Health Outcomes

Monique Ann-Marie Lynch and Geovanni Vinceroy Franklin

Abstract

WHO has defined health literacy as the degree to which individuals have the capacity to obtain, process and understand basic health information and services needed to make basic health decisions for themselves and their loved ones. The purpose of this article is to outline the scope of low health literacy as a concept and explore some appropriate interventions that researchers and healthcare professionals may use to reduce its negative impact on health outcomes such as mortality. The authors conclude by identifying areas of research that are needed to advance the conceptualization of health literacy in reducing hospital mortality and morbidity.

Keywords: health literacy, health promotion, health behavior, health knowledge, health outcomes

1. Background

Over the last decade, there have been many studies on a variety of interventions to decrease mortality by improving the health of patients through literacy. Some researchers such as [1] have addressed direct literacy related barriers primarily by testing interventions to make health education materials easier to understand. While other researchers like [2] have focused on indirect barriers by providing more general supportive interventions.

According to the [3] individuals with low to moderate health care, literacy skills face implications that may include the incompetence to carry out positive self-management, it also means higher medical costs due to more medication and treatment errors, more frequent hospitalizations, longer hospital stays, more visits to their health care provider, and a lack of necessary skills to obtain needed services.

Notwithstanding the colossal implications of low health literacy, there remains a significant amount of misunderstanding surrounding the concept and its implications for healthcare professionals and facilities in Jamaica [4]. Health literacy is not a new concept to the Jamaican healthcare community, however, it has not been a concept that is practiced on a daily basis in our facilities [4]. In other countries, it has caught the attention of researchers, policy makers, and healthcare professionals due to its prevalent impact on health and well-being.

The purpose of this chapter is to outline health literacy as a concept and explore some appropriate interventions that can assist researchers and healthcare professionals to reduce its negative impact on health outcomes such as mortality. The chapter will also address issues concerning low health literacy in developed and developing countries. Firstly, the major definitions of health literacy are

IntechOpen

presented in the introduction. Then, the description of interventions, how they have been applied, the challenges and outcomes, the discussion of resources required for implementation, the authors' unique perspective on the issue and proposed a framework for the implementation and evaluation of health literacy interventions, including culturally appropriate programming and the multi-disciplinary team approach.

2. Introduction

The term health literacy was introduced in 1974 in a paper calling for minimum health education standards for all grade-school levels in the United States (US) [5]. The World Health Organization (WHO) later defined health literacy as "the cognitive and social skills which determine the motivation and ability of individuals to gain access to, understand, and use information in ways that promote and maintain good health" [6].

Kirsch et al. [7] explained that the inability to read, write, and use numbers effectively, is common and is associated with a wide range of adverse health outcomes in the Caribbean and the Americas. There are five health outcomes of low health literacy, which are health knowledge, health behaviors, use of health care resources, intermediate markers of disease status, and measures of morbidity or mortality. However, this chapter will only focus on health knowledge and health behaviors because research indicates that knowledge affects behavioral outcomes [7]. Additionally, in order to reduce hospital mortality rates, individuals must have the knowledge base to obtain, process, and understand basic health information and services needed to make appropriate health decisions [8].

Health knowledge, or health education, refers to the knowledge and understanding people have about health-related issues [9]. It is important that people understand the causes of ill-health and recognize the extent to which they are vulnerable to, or at risk from, a health threat. The World Health Organization's (WHO) definition of health was expanded in 1996 as a state of complete physical, mental and social well-being and now includes a social dimension. Additionally, some social scientist of that era, believed that WHO expansion of the health, must include a spiritual dimension [10].

According to the aforementioned [11] definition of health, it summarized complete health as the development of the social, physical, mental and spiritual dimension of a person. These four aspects of health were highlighted in the Bible, by Jesus Christ, when he said in Luke 2 verse 52 "he (Jesus) increased in wisdom (mental health) and stature (physical health) in favor with God (spiritual health) and man (social health)," [12]. Therefore, in order for a person to experience complete health, there must be growth in these four dimensions. Individuals in this twenty-first century must know that impairment in any one of these dimensions will affect the proper function of the other dimensions. These four components of health knowledge, spiritual, mental, social and physical will be defined and discussed below.

2.1 Spiritual health

The term "spiritual intelligence" was coined by Danah Zohar in 1997. Additionally, Ken O'Donnell in 1997 who is an Australian author and consultant living in Brazil, also introduced the term "spiritual intelligence" and Michal Levin in 2000 use this "spiritual intelligence" in his book to draw attention to the concept of linking the spiritual and the material reality of life that is eventually concerned with the well-being of the universe and those who coexist in it [13–15].

It appears challenging to outwardly define spiritual health or spiritual intelligence without comprehending that the perception of spirituality is divergent from religiosity [16]. Fogel [17] opines that, for a very long time "spiritual" was, considered to be separate from "religious" and our secular societies prefers to steer as far as possible away from discussions on religion, for fear of kindling dormant conflicts or intruding on a taboo subject.

However, some researchers have tried to coin some functional definitions. For instance, [18] "spiritual intelligence is concerned with the inner life of mind and spirit and its relationship to being in the world." On the other hand, [19] defines spiritual intelligence as "the ability to act with wisdom and compassion, while maintaining inner and outer peace, regardless of the circumstances."

Research conducted by medical ethicists has reminded us that religion and spirituality form the basis of meaning and purpose for many people [20]. It is important to note that patients in health care institution, not only have the pain of physical ailment to confront with but the mental and spiritual pain that is associated with their sickness.

2.2 Mental health

According to [21], mental health literacy (knowledge) is defined as "knowledge and beliefs about mental disorders which aid their recognition, management or prevention." According to [22], there are key areas that help to equip persons with mental health knowledge. This will assist them with overcoming cultural and societal obstacles by challenging the fear of stigmatization. These areas include, but are not limited to; (a) the ability to recognize specific mental health problems, (b) knowledge and beliefs about risk factors, self-management approaches and the professional help available, (c) knowledge and beliefs about self-help interventions, (d) attitudes which facilitate recognition and appropriate help-seeking behaviors and (e) knowledge of how to seek and access mental health information.

The economic impacts of mental illness include its effects on personal income. These effects can only be quantified based on the ability of the persons with mental disorders or their caregivers to gauge the measurable economic burden of mental illness [23]. Bloom et al. [24] on the World Economic Forum (WEF) described three different approaches used to quantify economic disease burden, which do not only acknowledge the "hidden costs" of diseases, but also their impact on economic growth at a macroeconomic level (**Figure 1**).

Mental health is now getting a great deal of scrutiny around the world, it is an area of health that developing countries are seeking to end stigmatization and discrimination through literacy [26]. In a study conducted by [27] opines that the most commonly expressed emotional response to the mentally ill and mental illness was fear, often specifically a fear of "dangerousness." While the study reported some positive and empathetic responses, the most prominent emotional response was fear. Mental health literacy is the one of the most effective ways that fear towards the mentally challenged can be mitigated [28].

The possible recommendation could be that, to be effective and relevant, mental health educators must seek to improve individual literacy and numeracy skills. Furthermore, mental health information needs to be written clearly and the information must be accessible to those who need it. This type of information must be useful in improving practical social skills and the communicative elements should aid these persons to access and maintain health [29].

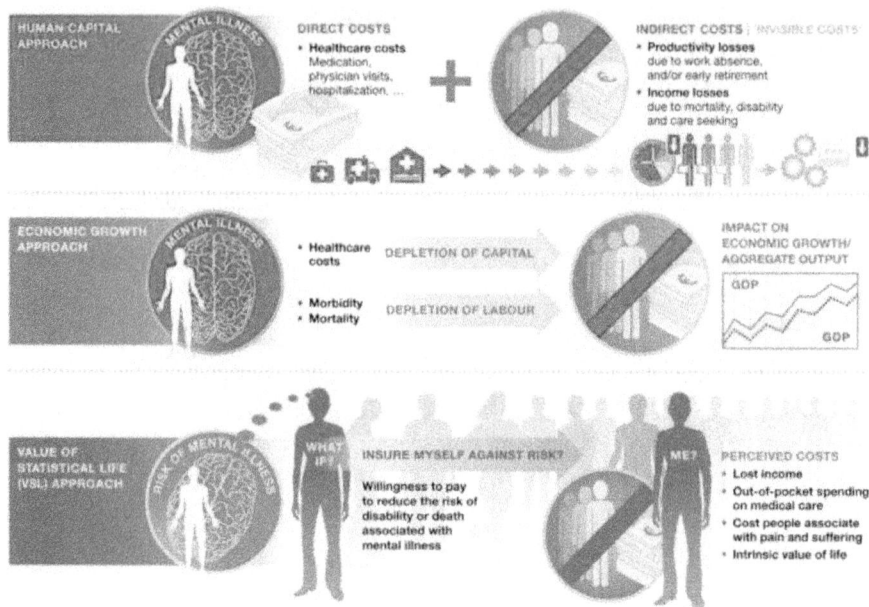

Figure 1.
Different approaches used to estimate economic costs of mental disorders [25].

2.3 Social health

The idea of social health is less recognizable to that of physical or mental health, but nonetheless, it's one of the four pillars (spiritual, mental and physical) that forms the WHO definitions of health. According to [30] accentuates that "a society is healthy when there is equal opportunity for all and access by all to the goods and services essential to full functioning as a citizen." Therefore, the success of a healthy society is influenced by the rule of law, equality in wealth distribution, public involvement in the decision-making process and a level of social capital.

In developing countries like Jamaica, there are many determinants of social health that affects the livelihood of many such as inequality, poverty, exploitation, violence and injustice, these are at the root of ill-health and the deaths of poor and marginalized people [31]. According to [32] mentioned that a determinant is any factor that contributes to person current state of health. Based on researchers, it is believed that social determinants of health are the situations in which people are born, grow, live, work and age. These conditions are molded base on the supply of money, power and resources at the global, national and local levels [33].

Julianne et al. [34] postulated that the quality of life and social relationship are closely related to mental health and the mortality rate. Furthermore, their opinion is that this modern way of life limits individual's social interactions, which results in people living insolation from extended families in developing countries. It is clear, that people of all different ages around the world are living alone, and loneliness on this crowded planet is becoming common [35].

2.4 Physical health

According to [36], physical health literacy is the ability to move with competence and confidence in a wide variety of physical activities in multiple environments that benefit the healthy development of the whole person. Moreover, it is supported by researchers that physical literacy is an essential and valuable human competency that can be described as a disposition learnt by human individuals surrounding that enthusiasm, confidence, physical competence, knowledge and understanding that establishes physical quests as an important part of their lifestyle [37].

In her research, [38] gave a summary of the key features of physical literacy:

- Everyone can be physically literate as it is appropriate to each individual's endowment,

- Everyone's physical literacy journey is unique, physical literacy is relevant and valuable at all stages and ages of life,

- The concept embraces much more than physical competence,

- At the heart of the concept is the motivation and commitment to be active, the disposition is evidenced by a love of being active, born out of the pleasure and satisfaction individuals experience in participation,

- A physically literate individual values and takes responsibility for maintaining purposeful physical pursuits throughout the life course and charting of progress of an individual's personal journey must be judged against previous achievements and not against any form of national benchmarks.

2.5 Health behaviors

There are several definitions for health behavior, one such researcher, [39] defined health behavior as the activity undertaken by people for the purpose of maintaining or enhancing their health, preventing health problems, or achieving a positive body image. Conner and Norman [40] added that any activity that is undertaken for the purpose of preventing or detecting disease or for improving health and wellbeing is defined as a health behavior. In the Handbook of Health Behavior Research, [41] defines health behavior as behavior patterns, actions and habits that relate to health maintenance, to health restoration and to health improvement' (Vol. 1, p. 3). Behaviors within this definition include medical service usage (e.g., physician visits, vaccination, screening), compliance with medical regimens (e.g., dietary, diabetic, antihypertensive regimens), and self-directed health behaviors (e.g., diet, exercise, smoking, alcohol consumption and illegal drug use).

It is common to differentiate health enhancing from health impairing behaviors. Institute of Medicine (US) Committee on Health and Behavior Research, Practice, and Policy [42] explained that health impairing behaviors have harmful effects on health or otherwise predispose individuals to diseases and even mortality. Such behaviors include smoking, excessive alcohol consumption, illegal drug misuse and high dietary fat and sugar consumption [42]. In contrast, [43] stated that engagement in health enhancing behaviors conveys health benefits or otherwise protect individuals from disease. Such behaviors include exercise, fruit and vegetable consumption, consumption of water instead of juice, limited alcohol consumption, no usage of illegal drugs and condom use in response to the threat of sexually transmitted diseases [43].

3. Methodology

This chapter utilized a multiple method approach to understand health literacy as an intervention to improve health outcomes. A meta-analysis, design was employed using three key phrase search and six keywords search resulting from the analysis of 43 articles. A breakdown of the methodologies using the two of the three key phrases is tabulated below (**Tables 1** and **2**).

Author	Population	Participants	Methods
[44]	One-third (77 million)	Over 19,000 adults from 38 states and the district of Columbia participated in the national and state-level assessments to create data for the NAAL.	The 2003 National Assessment of Adult Literacy (NAAL) which is a nationally representative assessment of English health literacy was distributed to American adults age 16 and older.

Table 1.
Showing key phrase: the relationship between health literacy and health outcomes.

Author	Population	Participants	Methods
[45]	Not stated	The demographic sample was 25 elderly and health illiterate persons using a mixed method and a convenience sampling approach.	The instrumentations used were verbal questioning (perception of drug visual aide assistance) and a written questionnaire on how prescription medication instructions should be written currently and in the future; since the sample was compiled of both literate and illiterate people, questions were asked verbally and the questionnaire was administered. The methods used were paper & pencil recording of the types of prescriptions each individual tool, what they should have taken and if they felt comfortable taking their current prescriptions.
[46]	Not stated	There were 15 studies dating from 1997 to 2006, a review confined to complex intervention study design was used and a sample range of 40-2046 participants.	A systematic review of randomized and quasi-randomized controlled trials with a narrative synthesis. The search strategy included searching eight databases from start date to 2007, reference checking and contacting expert informants. After the initial screen, two reviewers independently assessed eligibility, extracted data and evaluated study quality.
[47]	Not stated	There were 20 studies dating from 1992 to 2002, a controlled or uncontrolled experimental design was used and a sample range from 28 to 1744 participants.	The 20 studies were of three types: randomized controlled trials (n = 9), nonrandomized controlled trials (in which subjects were assigned to intervention or control groups by the day or the week or some other nonrandom fashion; n = 8), and uncontrolled, single-group trials (n = 3). The number of participants enrolled ranged from 28 to 1744; most studies had between 100 and 500 participants. All but 2 studies were conducted in the United States. Most interventions and outcome assessments were administered in single sessions. Interventions to improve dietary behavior and one other study delivered multisession interventions and/or followed participants longitudinally to assess changes in outcomes.

Table 2.
Showing key phrase: health literacy interventions to reduce mortality.

4. The relationship between health literacy and health outcomes

U.S. Department of Health and Human Services [8] explained in their research that low health literacy has been correlated with negative health outcomes, including reduced use of preventive health services, poor disease-specific outcomes for certain chronic conditions, and increased risk of hospitalization and mortality. Ad Hoc Committee on Health Literacy for the Council on Scientific Affairs, American Medical Association [48] agreed in their publication that health literacy is assumed to be a stronger predictor of health outcomes than social and economic status, education, gender, and age. With that being said, [49] stated that individuals with low health literacy have poorer health outcomes regardless of the illness they are diagnosed with. They went on to explain that low health literacy is more prevalent among vulnerable populations, such as the elderly, minorities, persons with lower education, and persons with chronic disease.

Several researches have shown that low literacy can have a direct and negative effect on health. Berkman et al. [50] explained that they expect this effect to be predominantly important for conditions that require substantial and complex self-care on the part of the patient because of the barriers to accessing and using health information, particularly written and calculated information. DeWalt et al. [2] agreed with [51, 48] by adding that low literacy can also be a marker for other conditions, such as poverty and lack of access to health care, that lead to poor health outcomes especially outcomes such as mortality.

The National Assessment of Adult Literacy report [44] explained that only 14% of adults have attained proficient health literacy, so in other words, nearly nine out of 10 adults may lack the skills needed to manage their health and prevent diseases. Additionally, it was reported that 16% of adults (50 million people) in having below basic health literacy and these adults were more likely to report their health as poorer (42%) than adults with proficient health literacy. Low literacy has been linked to poor health outcomes such as higher rates of hospitalization, less frequent use of preventive services and even hospital mortality [44].

4.1 Health literacy interventions to reduce mortality

4.1.1 The Jamaican context

In a study conducted by [45], a health literacy intervention was carried out in the cities of Black River, Balaclava, and Parottee, Jamaica by creating prescription drug visual aids that will assist the elderly health illiterate population with their medication adherence and to promote health literacy.

The results from the questionnaire used in the research showed that 80% of the overall sample were below the sixth-grade education literacy level, with 64% below the third-grade level and 16% between the fourth and sixth-grade levels. Additionally, 12% of respondents specifically from the city of Black River reported the ability to read but not to write. From the verbal questioning, 60% of the 64% of respondents who were below the third-grade education literacy level believed that visual aids would make medications easier to take. Furthermore, 8% of the 16% of respondents who were between the fourth and sixth grade education literacy levels believe that visual medication aides will benefit them. The results also displayed that a health literacy problem does exist in the areas in St. Elizabeth, Jamaica.

The findings indicated that the health literacy of the elderly population in rural Jamaica is a national health concern [45]. If these persons are incapable of understanding what type of medications they are taking and why, they are less likely to take them regularly and as scheduled/prescribed. However, many of these same persons understand and acknowledge that they also need help in terms of understanding and taking their medications and illnesses. The outcome of this study stated that rural elderly Jamaicans believe visual medication aides will benefit them and the results indicated that a health literacy problem does exist in the area, and visual aides are needed due to the literacy level and health literacy level of the region.

The main limitation stated for this intervention was that the sample size used was relatively small (25) and it might have played a role in respondents indicating their receptiveness to visual aids. Future implications of this research suggested that there is a need to conduct further research on the public health disparity between individuals in urban versus rural areas and that research might reveal disparities in the health outcomes.

4.1.2 The international context

Another study conducted by [46] in the United States of America, to evaluate the published literature of the effects of complex interventions intended to improve the health-related outcomes of individuals with limited literacy or numeracy. The focus of the 15 studies aforementioned in the methodology was on: health professionals (n = 2), literacy education (n = 1), and health education/management interventions (n = 12). In most of these studies (9 out 15), outcomes were measured in the intervention session or immediately afterwards. One study did not specify its follow-up period. The other five studies reported follow-up periods ranging from 1 week to 10.5 months with a median 5.5 months.

The primary results showed that there were statistically significant in 13/15 trials, though 8/13 had mixed results across primary outcomes. Two trials showed no significant positive finding in primary outcomes: one failed to show a significant improvement in health knowledge and the other failed to show significant changes in cholesterol and blood pressure changes. It was recommended that health related improvements were reported across all four intervention types, however, all interventions were complex interventions and it is not known which components of each initiative were effective. This, combined with the fact that some of the interventions were resource intensive, demands that future initiatives are carefully designed and based on sound theoretical and pragmatic reinforcements. The wider empowerment and community participation aspect of some of the interventions represent a welcome, broader approach to health literacy.

It was concluded that a variety of interventions for adults with limited literacy can be beneficial in improving some health outcomes especially mortality. The classes of outcome most likely to improve based on the study such as knowledge and self-efficacy. The implications suggested that more research was needed on the mechanisms of interventions that are most effective for improved health outcomes (specifically mortality). Additionally, there was limited evidence on interventions that targeted health professionals and their aptitude to deliver care optimally to patients with limited health literacy and to improve mortality rates especially in a hospital setting.

Pignone et al. [47] reported on a systematic review of interventions designed to improve health outcomes for persons with low health literacy in developed countries defined as United States, Canada, Western Europe, Japan, Australia and New Zealand. The focus of the studies were easy-to-read printed materials (n = 4), video/audio tapes (n = 4), computer-based programs (n = 3) and individual or group instructions (n = 9). The primary results displayed that the diversity of outcomes limits conclusions about the effectiveness, though effectiveness "appeared mixed". There were limitations in research quality that also hindered the drawing of conclusions. The five articles which dealt with the interaction between literacy level and the effect of the intervention stated mixed results. It is therefore recommended that research is needed to establish whether the correlation between low literacy and poor health outcomes is direct or indirect so as to most efficiently direct interventions.

The results of the interventions should be stratified by literacy level and future studies should focus on intermediate to longer term outcomes rather than short-term knowledge outcomes or health behaviors. There is no research which has considered how interventions may impact on health disparities or care costs based on race, ethnicity, culture or age. Multi-component interventions should be analyzed to establish efficacy and effectiveness.

It was concluded that several interventions based on the study have been developed to improve health for individual with low health literacy. There were limitations in the interventions tested and outcomes assessed make drawing deductions about effectiveness very difficult. Finally, advanced research is required to have a better understanding of the types of interventions that are most effective and efficient for overcoming health literacy-related barriers to good health and to improve health outcomes such as mortality.

World Health Organization Regional Office for South-East Asia [51] stated in their Health Literacy Toolkit for Low- and Middle-Income Countries that the Optimizing Health Literacy and Access to health information and services (Ophelia) approach is an effective system that supports the documentation of community health literacy needs, and the advancement and testing of possible solutions to reduce mortality. Each Ophelia project seeks to improve health and equity by increasing the availability and accessibility of health information and services in locally appropriate ways [51].

Projects have been carried out in Lavender Hill, an informal settlement, Cape Town: Ophelia South Africa under the title, "Identifying health literacy needs and developing local responses to health emergencies"; in Thailand under the title, "Optimizing health literacy needs of people" in Thailand and in New Zealand under the title, "Health literacy and Whanau Ora Outcomes: Ophelia New Zealand." The outcomes generated new data and tools that were used to inform practice and policy and aid practitioners at both the patient and organization levels to comprehend and meet the needs of the community, targeting those with low health literacy [52]. Batterham et al. [52] stated that the Ophelia approach is innovative as it recognizes that health literacy is multidimensional and different people may have different health literacy needs and that it took a systematic and grounded approach to intervention development.

4.2 Health literacy issues affecting developed and developing countries

In both developed and developing countries, a significant portion of the population has challenges in understanding health information which affect how they traverse the health care system. Decades of investigation show that there is a strong correlation between limited literacy in dealing with challenges in the health care and lower health knowledge intertwine with misinterpretation of prescriptions and lower receipt of preventive care [53].

In both developed and developing countries for the population to benefit from better health care, they must be knowledgeable about the various aspects of health care. Mayagah and Wayne [54] identified six general themes that help determine why health literacy is important for population health, firstly, large numbers of people affected because some developed countries have high adult literacy rates, while in developing countries approximately half have rates below the global developing country average of 79%. Research indicated that in developing countries literacy rates are lower among women than men, which is affecting how these persons respond to health information [55]. Additionally, difficulties with health literacy affect all people, but the elderly and chronically ill are most at-risk, and also have the greatest health care needs and expenses [56]. People with low health literacy are overwhelmed by health care because their skills and abilities are challenged by the demands and complexity required [57].

Secondly, poor health outcomes, findings indicated that there is a clear correlation between inadequate health literacy as measured by reading fluency and increased mortality rates. Report on the Council of Scientific Affairs [58] suggested that poor health literacy is "a stronger predictor of a person's health than age, income, employment status, education level, and race." Moreover, UNICEF, reported that hundreds of millions of people around the globe are living in extreme poverty. Both poverty and poor health are linked and can be the result of social, political, and economic injustices. The linkage is a vicious, self-perpetuating cycle where poverty causes poor health and poor health keeps communities in poverty. Research cited that people who are economically deprived and living in poor environments are faced with many health risk factors in their everyday life [59].

Thirdly, increasing rates of chronic disease are estimated to account for almost half (47%) of the total burden of disease. Likewise, chronic diseases often occur with co-morbidities (concomitant but unrelated diseases) and co-morbidity further increases the demand for health care. For example, individuals with diabetes and very high co-morbidity are expected to use 10 times the healthcare resources of the population average [60]. Research done on the Canadian Health Care System that indicated help is provided to people with chronic conditions such as diabetes, asthma, congestive heart failure, renal failure and chronic obstructive pulmonary disease. A large proportion of the available healthcare resources are devoted to treating chronic conditions and, in Canada, 67% of all health care costs are incurred as a result of caring for those with chronic conditions. More than half of Canadians aged 12 or older report at least one chronic condition and at age 65, 77% of men and 85% of women have at least one chronic condition [61]. Health literacy plays a crucial role in chronic disease self-management. In order to systematically manage chronic conditions on a daily basis, individuals must be able to assess, understand, evaluate, and use health information [62]. According to the Adult Literacy and Life Skills Survey, more than half (55%) of working-age Canadians do not have adequate levels of health literacy and only one in eight adults (12%) over age 65 has adequate health-literacy skills [63]. Also, [1] specified that populations most likely to experience low-literacy levels are among those being asked to manage their condition such as older adults, ethnic minorities, people with low levels of educational attainment, people with low income levels, nonnative speakers of English, and people with compromised health [64].

Also, those with low literacy skills are not likely to attend voluntary peer-led self-management programs even if they are aware, they exist. In 2003, the Institute of Medicine in its priority areas for national action, identified self-management/ health literacy as an area that cut across many health problems [64]. Schloman [65] opines that "improved health literacy was put forward as a condition necessary to enable active self-management of patients for most conditions."

Fourthly, health care costs; the additional costs of limited health literacy range from 3 to 5% of the total health care cost per year. Research has indicated that, insufficient health literacy has been associated with an increased need for disease management, higher medical service utilization among older, racial, ethnic minorities, and with low educational attainment [1]. Research conducted by the [66] in managing care, suggested that individuals with low health literacy have higher medical costs and are less efficient when using services than those individuals with adequate health literacy. Their findings estimated the costs associated with inadequate health literacy among adults at the national level to be $73 billion annually.

Fifthly, health information demand has created discrepancies between the reading levels of health-related materials and the reading skills of the intended audience. Often, the use of jargon and technical language made many health-related resources unnecessarily difficult to use [54]. The populations in both developing and developed countries are challenged with the increasing demands to understand and utilize health information, which are some of the complexities that are facing modern health care systems [67]. Additionally, the increasing proportion of people living with chronic conditions, competencies for proactive self-management of health and participation in collaborative care have become key public health agendas. The ability to take active part in shared decision making with healthcare providers is important for adherence to treatment, self-management of chronic diseases [68].

Lastly, equity is a factor that suggests that low levels of health literacy often means that a person is unable to manage their own health effectively, access health services effectively, and understand the information available to them and thus make informed healthy decisions [54]. Researchers over the past two decades, have been investigating the importance of health literacy and have examined over 1600 related research articles such as the field of "health care disparities" [69]. Improving the health literacy of those with the worst health outcomes is an important tool in reducing health inequalities [54].

It's evident that the challenges with [70] equity may still exist today. Many countries have failed to document data about the population that will make inferences about the disparities that have contributed to the lower quality of care. Due to the limited data about these disparities, situations that affects individuals with low literary skills are often times overlooked and efforts to address inequities in health care are rendered as ineffective. Furthermore, health care researchers are of the view that data to properly assess these disparities can be collected. However, health care organizations are lacking in the measurement tools to assess patient literacy in populations served by operating health care systems [70]. Isham [70] further lamented that quality measures for improving health literacy are lacking. Therefore, the current problems of low health literacy should perhaps be viewed less as a patient problem and more as a challenge to health care providers and health systems to reach out and more effectively communicate with patients. The United Nations Educational, Scientific and Cultural Organization (UNESCO) Institute of Statistics (UIS) projected that over 776 million adults, which is about 16% of the world's adult population lacking basic literacy skills [71]. These figures appear to be alarmed by the strides that the human race has made in development of education. Additionally, a recent survey of health literacy among 2000 adults in the United Kingdom found that one in five people had difficulty with the basic skills required for understanding simple information that could lead to better health [72].

It seems that quality health care is advancing in the developed countries due to the developments in technology [73], while on the other hand, the population in developing countries is affected by low literacy levels due to the limited advancement of technology [74]. However, research has indicated that 60% of adult Canadians (ages 16 and older) lack the capacity to obtain, understand and act on health information and services, and also the ability to make appropriate health decisions on their own. In addition, the proportion of adults with low levels of health literacy is significantly higher among certain groups. These findings raise questions of equity [54].

Findings from comparable studies done in Europe, Australia, Latin America and other countries have correlated literacy levels with access to education, ethnicity and age as determinants to better health care [75]. Other studies have indicated that having limited literacy or numeracy skills also acts as an independent risk factor for poor health, which lead to medication errors and insufficient understanding of diseases and treatments [76]. Additionally, [49] from their review determined that there is a relationship between literacy and health outcomes that was directly corresponding to several adverse health-related factors, such as, knowledge about health and health care, hospitalization, global measures of health, and some chronic diseases.

In exploring the link between literacy and mortality, Baker and colleagues suggest that there is a strong correlation between inadequate health literacy—as measured by reading fluency—and increased mortality rates [77]. Neuroscience and Behavioral Health specialists opine that health literacy is essential to overall patient care. It's very important for every citizen in both developed and developing countries to understand basic health information. This understanding will empower people to make better decision as it relates to self-care and medical decisions. Educating the population of any country about health is crucial in mitigating inequalities that exist in health care systems. It is evident that individuals with low health literacy have poorer health status and higher rates of hospital admission, are less likely to adhere to prescribed treatments and care plans, experience more drug and treatment errors, and make less use of preventive services [78].

Poor health literacy with limited access to education may result in a deficiency in patient self-management. According to [79] believes that lack of understanding of procedures of basic health information, will interfere with their ability to take better care of themselves and make health related informed decisions. Therefore, it's evident that patients who are involved self-management will mostly experience positive health outcomes and place fewer demands on the healthcare system.

The role of healthcare facilities and health care professionals is to assist patients in becoming better in self-management and limit the patients' dependency on the health care system. It's important to understand that health literacy is pivotal in the management of chronic medical conditions. Patients need to learn and understand self-management by having access to health information which will enable them to better cope with daily challenges (includes a complex medical regimen, plan and make lifestyle adjustment) that comes with chronic illness [80].

Another major issue that affects both developed and developing countries is the cost that is attached to health care. Research has concluded that is difficult to correctly evaluate the real economic cost that is associated with low health literacy. Factors such as what constitutes health literacy and insufficient data collection on the frequency of low literacy help to compound the challenge of economic cost. Researchers believe that despite these challenges in evaluating the impact of limited health literacy studies that are available underscore the importance of addressing limited health literacy from a financial perspective [81].

Vernon et al. [82] revealed that the findings of a health literacy cost study that was based on an analysis of US National data revealed that the cost of low health literacy to the U.S. economy is in the range of $106–$238 billion annually. Additionally, he stated, "when one accounts for the future costs of low health literacy that result from current actions (or lack of action), the real present-day cost of low health literacy is closer in range to $1.6–$3.6 trillion" [82].

It is clear that tracking the economic cost associated with low health literacy will strongly depend on the strength of the economic status of the developed and developing countries. Rootman and Ronson [83] stated that inequality is another major factor that affects the citizens of all countries. They postulate that "a person's literacy level is influenced by many factors and conditions; these determinants of literacy are similar to the determinants of health commonly referred to in the health promotion literature." Studies have indicated that factors like education, personal ability, early childhood development, aging, living and working conditions, gender and culture and language help to influence literacy rates in countries around the world [83].

Research in the United Kingdom indicated [84] that low health literacy is emphatically connected with more unfortunate health outcomes, and every dynamic increment towards higher health literacy is related to a more prominent probability of participating in a solid and healthier way of life, explicitly eating at least five servings of fruits and vegetables and being a non-smoker. Likewise, [83] expressed that low levels of health literacy frequently imply that an individual cannot deal with their own wellbeing adequately, access health services viably, or comprehend the data accessible to them and therefore settle on educated and sound health choices. Enhancing the health literacy of those with the poor, negative health outcomes is a critical device in diminishing health inequalities [83].

It's important for developing countries to comprehend that health literacy entails development of individual level of knowledge, personal skills and the confidence to take action to improve self-management and community health by encouraging changes in the personal lifestyle and living conditions. Therefore, health literacy is more than people reading pamphlets and making appointments but is the overall improvement in the individual's ability to access health data and their capacity to effectively use that information [85].

In both developed and developing countries but mostly in developing nations, health care systems need to address the needs of communities and breaking down the barriers that exist through health literacy, such as, lack of compliance medication regime. Lack of health educators working with vulnerable citizens in communities like women, those living rural areas and immigrants. Other barriers like language, socio-political, economic and cultural barriers and time constraints pose challenges to health care providers and health literacy advancement. Research has shown that these vulnerable people have significantly worse outcomes which is associated with high mortality and morbidity rates due to the lack health literacy levels. Therefore, developing countries like the Caribbean in tackling the economic cost of low literacy must apply a comprehensive, and integrated health approach to the services that are important in transforming in the model of care [79].

Pan American Health Organization [79] reported that regardless of the improvements has been achieved in health literacy, poverty and inequities remain a challenge in the Region. Recent data suggest that Latin America and the Caribbean (LAC) remains the most inequitable region in the world, with 29% of the population below the poverty line and the poorest 40% of the population receiving less than 15% of total income. Such inequities are reflected in health outcomes: for example, the Region of the Americas did not achieve the Millennium Development Goal (MDG) target for the reduction of maternal mortality by 2015, and despite significant reductions in infant mortality, very sharp differences exist between countries. Without specific interventions to transform health systems, economic growth is not sufficient to reduce inequities.

As a developing country, Jamaica is confronted with many health issues. Specifically, there are concerns with an ever-aging population, which continues to grow in size at an astounding rate of 11.3% each year [86]. Coverson [45] asked these impertinent questions, "who will take care of this aging population, what services will be available, and how the elderly will maintain a reasonable quality of life are all questions that are facing Jamaica in the near future. People are living longer and with this increase in life-years come other concerns such as the cost of care, who will administer the care, and access to care as travel becomes more difficult with increased age."

Paul and Bourne [87] suggested that this vulnerable group in the population that are affected by reading difficulties have greater challenges in understanding the high level of grammar associated with health care instruments, diagnostic tests, directions and medications. This lack of comprehension can result in patients experiencing confusion in navigating the healthcare system, and are significantly handicapped in the task of self-management or caring for their family members.

4.3 Cultural issues affecting health literacy in developed and developing countries

Baker [88] concurring with other researchers agree that culturally, health care is multifaceted idea. National Center for Cultural Competence [89], culture has been defined as the "integrated pattern of human behavior that includes thoughts, communications, actions, customs, beliefs, values and institutions of a racial, ethnic, religious or social group."

State of illness is viewed through a cultural lens in countries around the world. With these cultural lens people summarize health and sickness and based on their perception will respond to the health message. It's important to note that culture will help people determine what treatment options are best (by going to the medical doctor or the herbalist), and it helps people interpret symptoms [90]. It is important to recognize that based on these cultural health beliefs that an individual has, will greatly impact how they think and feel about their health and health challenges. It also affects the kind of people that they seek care from and how they respond to recommendations to make changes to their lifestyle and how they accept health intervention messages [91].

Due the complex nature of health literacy and cultural practices, health literacy cannot have one "sprang" approach in reaching the populace. Health literacy is not determined solely by an individual's capacity to read, understand, process, and act on health information. However, it's dependent on the request that individuals make for health information and their ability to decode, interpret, and understand the information presented. Furthermore, health literacy is not constant, but is a dynamic state that may change with the situation [88]. Researchers have agreed that in order to effectively deal with low health literacy in the health care system, there needs to be an aggressive research agenda that will in cooperate evidence base tools that will provide relevant data in order to address these challenges [92].

Cultures also vary in their styles of communication, in the meaning of words and gestures, and even in what can be discussed regarding the body, health, and illness. Health literacy requires communication and mutual understanding between patients and their families and healthcare providers and staff. Culture and health literacy, both influences the content and outcomes of health care encounters [29]. Cooper and Roter [93] review the relationship that exists between the relationship between culture, patient-provider interaction, and quality of care and have concluded that culture gives significance to health information and messages. The awareness that people have about the definitions of health and illness, preferences, language and cultural barriers, and stereotypes are strongly influenced by the individual's culture which can greatly sway health literacy and health outcomes. Furthermore, others challenges are developed due to the different educational backgrounds among patients and providers and those responsible to create health information can lead to cultural challenges based on the wording used to share the information [93].

Research done on the importance of culture and health literacy in European-American cultural groups indicated that the use of language differs in discussing symptoms such as pain [94–95]. Base on the cultural, linguistic differences were linked with changes in diagnoses, regardless of symptomology. African-American patients frequently experience shorter physician-patient interactions and less patient-centered visits than Caucasian patients [93, 96].

With the ever increasing melting pot of ethnicity in countries around the world, health care systems are forced to recognize these different ethnic groups with cultural diversity in order to be inclusive [93]. Therefore, cultural, social, and family norms have transformed the attitudes and beliefs which will significantly impact the levels of health literacy (native language, socioeconomic status, gender, race, and ethnicity are considered as influencers that limits person's control which affects his or her ability to participate fully in a health-literate society [97]. It behooves the health care providers to properly utilize the various modes of communication such as news publishing, advertising, marketing, and the plethora of health information sources available through electronic channels are also integral to the social-cultural landscape of health literacy when communicating with cultural masses [29].

By incorporating a greater focus on health literacy, health care professionals will move closer toward a patient-centered health care system (**Figures 1** and **2**).

Governments around the world must understand that need to develop a health care system that works is not the burden of health care consumer. The need to improve health literacy must be seen as a partnership between public and private organizations whose primary focus is to help citizens become health literate. This cohesive partnership will help both developed and developing nation's realized improvements in health literacy will play a major role in improving health care systems and the holistic health for their citizens [73].

Since health literacy is not constant, but dynamic, governments must observe health literacy as fundamental to health, and essential for improving quality of patient care. Low levels of health literacy present a formidable challenge to the widespread and effective use of patient self-management [99]. However, these challenges can be met. Although, health literacy continues to get more attention at the national level and economic cost becomes visible, improving health literacy will be crucial in reducing adverse outcomes that are connected with low health literacy [73]. Within the twenty-first century there is no universal solution, but by gathering relevant data and implementing best practices can be strategies that can be steadily used to improve health literacy for populations around the world. By simplifying health literacy information which will increase the usability of this information must be the priority focus.

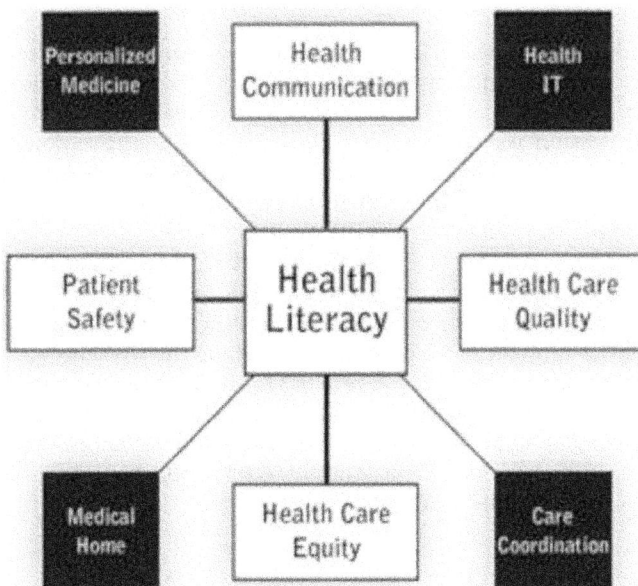

Figure 2.
The intersection of health literacy with health care improvement [98].

When patients can relate health information in plain language in both the written and spoken formats will help in improving the decision-making capacity of the client [92]. The method of assessing and responding to health literacy at the governmental level has been a progression in the focus of health literacy as a responsibility of the patient. However, organizations and systems are accountable for designing service delivery that challenges the health literacy needs of the clients of health care providers [99].

5. Recommendations

Governments, policy makers, organizations, health practitioners and community members must work in partnership to address health literacy issues contributing to poor health outcomes such as mortality and morbidity. We are therefore recommending the following:

- Implementing the Ophelia (Optimizing Health Literacy and Access to health information and services) Australian approach in our health care system and in extent in all developing countries. This approach involves the collaboration of a wide range of healthcare professionals, government leaders or representatives, community health center or hospital patients and leaders to develop health literacy interventions that are based on needs identified within a hospital or community.

- Develop and implement policies that promote documentation of health literacy issues and the implementation of targeted responses.

- Develop and implement policies that promote equitable access to health information and services for all citizens.

6. Conclusions

This visualization for health literacy as an intervention to reduce hospital mortality and morbidity rates can be effective as the data presented shows the importance of meeting the needs of patients with low health literacy in Jamaica. Healthcare professionals have an important role to play, but the responsibility for achieving real progress for patients facing challenges related to health literacy must extend to greater government involvement by creating health literacy policies and programs in both rural and urban areas.

Greater emphasis needs to be placed where the hard-to-reach or disadvantaged or vulnerable groups which include the elderly, children and patients with disability (mental/physical/intellectual). In Jamaica, we are still stuck at the developmental stage of understanding the scope of health literacy and the challenges patients face and developing cultural relevant interventions to address them. The relationship between health literacy and health outcomes such as mortality and morbidity needs to be explored through further research. The interventions identified in this chapter are stepping stones which need significantly greater support, resources for research and implementation of interventions.

Author details

Monique Ann-Marie Lynch[1*] and Geovanni Vinceroy Franklin[2]

1 World Federation for Mental Health, University of the West Indies, Mona

2 University of the West Indies, Mona

*Address all correspondence to: monique.a.lynch@gmail.com

IntechOpen

References

[1] Nielsen-Bohlman L, Panzer AM, Kindig DA. Health Literacy: A Prescription to End Confusion. The National Academies Press; 2004. Available from: http://www.nap.edu/ books/ 0309091179/html/

[2] DeWalt DA, Broucksou KA, Hawk V, Brach C, Hink A, Rudd R, et al. Developing and testing the health literacy universal precautions toolkit. Nursing Outlook. 2011;59(2):85-94. DOI: 10.1016/j.outlook.2010.12.002

[3] Office of Disease Prevention and Health Promotion. Health Literacy and Health Outcomes. 2004. Available from: https://health.gov/communication/ literacy/quickguide/factsliteracy.htm

[4] Campbell W. Health Literacy Key for All Jamaicans. 2017. Available from: http://jamaica-gleaner. com/article/letters/20170218/ health-literacy-key-all-jamaicans

[5] U.S. Department of Health and Human Services. Healthy People 2010. Washington, DC: U.S. Government Printing Office; 2000. Originally developed for Ratzan SC, Parker RM. Introduction. In: Selden CR, Zorn M, Ratzan SC, Parker RM, editors. National Library of Medicine Current Bibliographies in Medicine: Health Literacy. NLM Pub. No. CBM 2000-1. Bethesda, MD: National Institutes of Health, U.S. Department of Health and Human Services; 2000

[6] World Health Organization (WHO). Health Promotion Glossary. Division of Health Promotion, Education and Communications Health Education and Health Promotion Unit. Geneva: World Health Organization; 1998. p. 10. Available from: www.who.int/hpr/NPH/ docs/hp_glossary_en.pdf

[7] Kirsch I, Jungeblut A, Jenkins L, Kolstat A. Adult Literacy in America:

A First Look at the Findings of the National Adult Literacy Survey. 2000. pp. 1-201

[8] U.S. Department of Health and Human Services. Quick Guide to Health Literacy Services. 2011. Available from: http://www.health.gov/communication/ literacy/quickguide/factsbasic.html

[9] Donatelle R. Promoting healthy behavior change. In: Health: The Basics. 8th ed. San Francisco, CA: Pearson Education, Inc.; 2009. p. 4

[10] World Health Organization. Constitution of the World Health Organization—Basic Documents. 45th ed. Switzerland: WHO Press; 2006. Available from: https:// www.who.int/governance/eb/ who_constitution_en.pdf

[11] World Health Organization, Geneva. Equity in Health and Health Care. 1996. Available from: www.WHO/ ARA/96.1

[12] Vaughan, F. What is Spiritual Intelligence? Journal of Humanistic Psychology. Sage Publications. 2003;42(2):16-33

[13] Zohar D. Rewiring the Corporate Brain: Using the New Science to Rethink How We Structure and Lead Organizations. Berrett-Koehler Publishers; 1997. ISBN: 9971-5-1214-9

[14] O'Donnell K. Endoquality—As dimensões emocionais e espirituais do ser humano nas organanizões. Brazil: Casa da Qualidade; 1997. ISBN 858565127X

[15] Levin M. Spiritual Intelligence. Australia: Hodder Headline Publishers; 2000. ISBN 0-340-73394-2

[16] Koenig HG, McCullough M, Larson DB. The Handbook of Religion and

Health. New York: Oxford University
Press; 2000

[17] Fogel RW. The Fourth Great
Awakening and the Future of
Egalitarianism. Chicago: The University
of Chicago Press; 2000

[18] Vaughan F. What is spiritual
intelligence? Journal of Humanistic
Psychology. 2003;**42**(2):16-33

[19] Wigglesworth C. Why spiritual
intelligence is essential to mature
leadership. Integral Leadership Review.
2006;**VI**(3):224-227

[20] Foglio JP, Brody H. Holy religion,
faith and family medicine. The Journal
of Family Practice. 1988;**27**(5):473-474

[21] Jorm AF, Korten AE, Jacomb PA.
'Mental health literacy': A survey of
the public's ability to recognise mental
disorders and their beliefs about the
effectiveness of treatment. Medical
Journal of Australia. 1997;**166**:182-186

[22] Public Health England. Local Action
on Health Inequalities; Promoting
Health Literacy to Reduce Health
Inequalities. London: Public Health
England; 2015

[23] World Health Organization, Geneva.
Investing in Mental Health. 2003.
Available from: https://www.who.int/
mental_health/media/investing_mnh.pdf

[24] Bloom DE, Cafiero ET, Jané-Llopis
E, Abrahams-Gessel S, Bloom LR,
Fathima S, et al. The Global Economic
Burden of Noncommunicable Diseases.
Geneva: World Economic Forum; 2011

[25] Traurmann S, Rehm J, Wittchen
H-U. The Economic Costs of Mental
Disorders. 2016. Available from: embor.
embopress.org/content/early/2016/08/04/
embr.201642951.figures/only

[26] World Health Organization. Mental
Health: A Call for Action by World

Health Ministers. 2001. Available from:
https://www.who.int/mental_health/
media/en/249.pdf

[27] Hickling FW, Arthur CM,
Robertson-Hickling H, Haynes-Robinson
T, Abel W, Whitley R. Mad, sick, head
nuh good: Mental illness stigma in
Jamaican communities. Transcultural
Psychiatry. 2010;**47**:252-275

[28] Academies of Sciences, Engineering,
and Medicine. Approaches to Reducing
Stigma. In: Ending Discrimination
against People with Mental and
Substance Use Disorders: The Evidence
for Stigma Change. Washington, DC:
National Academies Press (US); 2016.
Available from: https://www.ncbi.nlm.
nih.gov/books/NBK384914/

[29] Nutbeam D. Health literacy as
a public health goal: A challenge for
contemporary health education and
health communication strategies into
the 21st century. Health Promotion
International. 2000;**15**(3):259-267

[30] Russell RD. Social health: An
attempt to clarify this dimension of
well-being. International Journal of
Health Education. 1973;**16**:74-82

[31] People's Health Movement. People's
Charter for Health. 2018. Available from:
https://phmovement.org/wp-content/
uploads/2018/06/phm-pch-english.pdf

[32] U.S. Department of Health and
Human Services. Healthy People 2020
Draft. U.S. Government Printing Office.
2009

[33] World Health Organization.
"Closing the Gap in a Generation:
Health Equity Through Action on the
Social Determinants of Health" The
Final Report of the WHO Commission
on Social Determinants of Health.
Switzerland: WHO Press; 2008.
Available from: https://www.who.int/
social_determinants/final_report/
csdh_finalreport_2008.pdf

[34] Julianne H, Smith T, Bradley Layton J. Social relationships and mortality risk: A meta-analytic review. PLoS Medicine. 2010;7(7):1-2

[35] Klinenberg E. Social isolation loneliness, and living alone: Identifying the risks for public health. American Journal of Public Health. 2016;**106**(5):786-787. Available from: https://www.ncbi.nlm.nih.gov/pmc/articles/PMC4985072/

[36] Mandigo J, Francis N, Lodewyk K, Lopez R. Physical literacy for educators. Physical Education and Health Journal. 2012;**75**(3):27-30

[37] Almond L, Whitehead M. Physical literacy: Clarifying the nature of the concept. Physical Education Matters. 2012;**7**(1):255-257. ISSN: 1751-0988

[38] Whitehead M. Physical Literacy: Throughout the Lifecourse. London: Routledge; 2010

[39] Cockerham WC. Medical Sociology. 12th ed. Boston: Pearson Education; 2012. p. 120

[40] Conner M, Norman P, editors. Predicting Health Behaviour. Buckingham, UK: Open University Press; 1996

[41] Gochman DS, editor. Handbook of Health Behavior Research. Vol. 1-4. New York, NY: Plenum; 1997

[42] Institute of Medicine (US) Committee on Health and Behavior Research, Practice, and Policy. Health and Behavior: The Interplay of Biological, Behavioral, and Societal Influences, Behavioral Risk Factors. Vol. 3. Washington, DC: National Academies Press; 2001. Available from: https://www.ncbi.nlm.nih.gov/books/NBK43744/

[43] Conner MT. Health Behaviors. 2002. Available from:

https://www.researchgate.net/publication/266862660_Health_Behaviors

[44] National Center for Education Statistics. The Health Literacy of America's Adults: Results From the 2003 National Assessment of Adult Literacy. Washington, DC: U.S. Department of Education; 2006

[45] Coverson D. Health literacy in rural Jamaica: Visual aides to assist and increase medication adherence. MOJ Public Health. 2015;**2**(5):149-152. DOI: 10.15406/mojph.2015.02.00038

[46] Clement S, Ibrahim S, Crichton N, Wolf M, Rowlands G. Complex interventions to improve the health of people with limited literacy: A systematic review. Patient Education and Counseling. 2009;**75**(3):340-351

[47] Pignone M, DeWalt DA, Sheridan S, Berkman N, Lohr KN. Interventions to improve health outcomes for patients with low literacy. Journal of General Internal Medicine. 2005;**20**:185-192

[48] Ad Hoc Committee on Health Literacy for the Council on Scientific Affairs, American Medical Association. Health Literacy: Report of the Council on Scientific Affairs. JAMA. 1999;**281**(6):552-557. DOI:10.1001/jama.281.6.552

[49] DeWalt DA, Berkman ND, Sheridan SL, Lohr KN, Pignone M. Literacy and health outcomes: A systematic review of the literature. Journal of General Internal Medicine. 2004;**19**:1228-1239

[50] Berkman ND, Dewalt DA, Pignone MP. (RTI International-University of North Carolina Evidence-based Practice Center): Literacy and Health Outcomes: Evidence Report/Technology Assessment Number. 2004. Available from: http://www.ahrq.gov/clinic/litinv.htm

[51] World Health Organization Regional Office for South-East Asia. Health

Literacy Toolkit for Low- and Middle-Income Countries that the Optimizing Health Literacy and Access to Health Information and Services. 2014. Available from: http://www.searo.who.int/entity/healthpromotion/documents/hl_tookit/en/

[52] Batterham R, Buchbinder R, Beauchamp A, Dodson S, Elsworth GR, Osborne RH. The Optimising HEalth LIterAcy (Ophelia) process: Study protocol for using health literacy profiling and community engagement to create and implement health reform. 2014. Available from: https://bmcpublichealth.biomedcentral.com/articles/10.1186/1471-2458-14-694

[53] Adult Basic and Literacy Education Inter-agency Coordinating Council. A Report on Health Literacy. Pennsylvania State University. 2002. Available from: http://www.csg.org/knowledgecenter/docs/ToolKit03HealthLiteracy.pdf

[54] Mayagah K, Wayne M. Promoting Health and Development: Closing the Implementation Gap. World Health Organization Report, Nairobi, Kenya; 2009. pp. 26-30

[55] Lam Y, Broaddus ET, Surkan PJ. Literacy and healthcare-seeking among women with low educational attainment: Analysis of cross-sectional data from the 2011 Nepal demographic and health survey. International Journal for Equity in Health. 2013;**12**:95. DOI: 10.1186/1475-9276-12-95

[56] Chesser AK, Keene Woods N, Smothers K, Rogers N. Health literacy and older adults: A systematic review. Gerontology & Geriatric Medicine. 2016;**2**:1-13. DOI: 10.1177/2333721416630492

[57] Kutner M, Greenberg E, Jin Y, Paulsen C. The Health Literacy of America's Adults: Results From the 2003

National Assessment of Adult Literacy (NCES 2006-483). Washington, DC: U.S. Department of Education, National Center for Education Statistics; 2006

[58] Ad Hoc Committee on Health Literacy for the Council on Scientific Affairs, American Medical Association. Health Literacy: Report of the Council on Scientific Affairs. JAMA. 1999;**281**(6):562-564. DOI:10.1001/jama.281.6.562

[59] Amini S. Poor Health Outcomes Associated with Low SES Status; How Poverty Can Be a Determinant of Health. University of Florida(UF) Health; 2016

[60] Broemeling A-M, Watson D, Black C. Chronic Conditions and Co-Morbidity Among Residents of British Columbia. Vancouver, BC: Centre for Health Services and Policy Research; 2005. Available from: https://www.researchgate.net/publication/255585868_Chronic_conditions_and_co-morbidity_among_residents_of_British_Columbia

[61] Gilmour H, Park J. Dependency, chronic conditions and pain in seniors. Health Reports. 2006;**16**(supplement):21-32. Statistics Canada catalogue no. 82-003-SIE

[62] van der Heide I, Poureslami I, Mitic W, Shum J, Rootman I, Mark Fitz Gerald J. Health literacy in chronic disease management: A matter of Interaction. Journal of Clinical Epidemiology. 2018;**2**:134-138

[63] Canadian Council on Learning. State of Learning in Canada: No Time for Complacency. Canadian Council on Learning; 2007. Available from: https://www.dartmouthlearning.net/wp-content/uploads/2013/02/State-of-Learning-in-Canada-No-Time-for-Compacency-2007.pdf

[64] Current Clinical Issues. The crucial link between literacy and health. Annals

of Internal Medicine. 2003;**139**(10):875-878. DOI: 10.7326/0003-4819-139-10-200311180-00038

[65] Schloman B. Health literacy: A key ingredient for managing personal health. Online Journal of Issues in Nursing. 2004;**9**(2):6

[66] Center on an Aging Society at Georgetown University. Low Health Literacy Skills Increase Annual Health Care Expenditures by $73 Billion. Center on an Aging Society at Georgetown University. 1999. Available from: https://hpi.georgetown.edu/healthlit/

[67] Bodenheimer T, Lorig K, Holman H, Grumbach K. Patient self-management of chronic disease in primary care. Journal of the American Medical Association. 2002;**288**(19):2469-2475

[68] Appelbaum PS. Review clinical practice. Assessment of patients' competence to consent to treatment. The New England Journal of Medicine. 2007;**357**(18):1834-1840

[69] Institute of Medicine. Unequal Treatment: Confronting Racial and Ethnic Disparities in Healthcare. Washington, DC: The National Academies Press; 2003

[70] Isham G. Opportunity at the Intersection of Quality Improvement, Disparities Reduction, and Health Literacy, Toward Health Care Equity and Patient-Centeredness. Institute of Medicine Workshop Summary. 2009

[71] UNESCO. 2009. Available from: http://www.unesco.org/en/efa-international-coordination/the-efa-movement/efagoals/adult-literacy/27

[72] Sihota S, Lennard L. Health lLiteracy: Being able to make the most of health. In: National Consumer Council. 2004

[73] Koh HK, Berwick DM, Clancy CM, et al. New federal policy initiatives to boost health literacy can help the nation move beyond the cycle of costly 'crisis care'. Health Aff (Millwood). 2012;**31**(2):434-443. DOI:10.1377/hlthaff.2011.1169

[74] Mia M, Omar A. Technology Advancement in Developing Countries During Digital Age. 2012. Available from: https://pdfs.semanticscholar.org/22b7/52250e726faefd35c64d8836328533bc4c42.pdf

[75] Health literacy Australia. Australian Bureau of Statistics. 2006. Available from: http://www.ausstats.abs.gov.au/ausstats/subscriber.nsf/0/73ED158C6B14BB5ECA2574720011AB83/$File/42330_2006.pdf

[76] Williams MV, Baker DW, Parker RM, Nurss JR. Relationship of functional health literacy to patients' knowledge of their chronic disease: A study of patients with hypertension and diabetes. Archives of Internal Medicine. 1998;**158**:166-172

[77] Baker DW, Parker RM, Williams MV, Clark WS. Health literacy and the risk of hospital admission. Journal of General Internal Medicine. 1998;**13**:791-800

[78] Board on Neuroscience and Behavioral Health, Institute of Medicine. Health Literacy: A Prescription to End Confusion. Washington, DC: National Academies Press; 2004

[79] Pan American Health Organization. Regional declaration on the new orientation for primary health care (Declaration of Montevideo), 46th Directing Council, 57th Session of the Regional Committee, Washington, D.C., Sept. 26-30 (CD46/13). 2005

[80] Johnston Lloyd L, Ammary N, Epstein L, Johnson R, Rhee K. A trans disciplinary approach to improve health

literacy and reduce disparities. Health Promotion Practice. 2006;**3**:331-335

[81] Institute of Medicine. Health Literacy: A Prescription to End Confusion. 2004. Available from: http://www.iom.edu/?id=19750

[82] Vernon JA, Trujillo A, Rosenbaum S, DeBuono B. Low Health Literacy: Implications for National Health Policy. Washington, DC: Department of Health Policy, School of Public Health and Health Services, The George Washington University; 2007

[83] Rootman I, Ronson B. Literacy and Health in Canada: What We Have Learned and What Can Help in the Future? 2003. Available from: http://www.cpha.ca/uploads/portals/h-l/literacy_e.pdf

[84] Schwartzberg JG, Cowett A, Vangeest J, Wolf MS. Communication techniques for patients with low health literacy: A survey of physicians, nurses and pharmacists. American Journal of Health Behavior. 2007;**31**(Suppl 1):S96-S104

[85] UN Chronicle. Health Literacy and Sustainable Development. The Magazine of the United Nation. 2009;**XLXI**(1&2).p. 1

[86] World Health Organization. Definition of an Older or Elderly Person. Geneva: 2014. Available from: https://www.who.int/healthinfo/survey/ageingdefnolder/en/

[87] Paul A, Bourne CM. Health literacy and health seeking behavior among older men in a middle income nation. Patient Related Outcome Measures. 2010;**2010**:39-49

[88] Baker DW. The meaning and the measure of health literacy. Journal of General Internal Medicine. 2006;**21**(8):878-883

[89] National Center for Cultural Competence. Cultural Competence. Center for Child and Human Development: Georgetown University; 1989. Available from: https://nccc.georgetown.edu/curricula/culturalcompetence.html

[90] Heurtin-Roberts S, Reisin E. The relation of culturally influenced lay models of hypertension to compliance with treatment. American Journal of Hypertension. 1992;**5**(11):787-792

[91] Morse A. Language access: Helping non-english speakers navigate health and human services. In: National Conference of State Legislature's Children's Policy Initiative; 2003

[92] DeWalt DA, Callahan LF, Hawk VH, Broucksou KA, Hink A, Rudd R, et al. Health Literacy Universal Precautions Toolkit. (AHRQ Publication No. 10-0046-EF). Rockville, MD: Agency for Healthcare Research and Quality; 2010

[93] Cooper LA, Roter DL. Patient-provider communication: The effect of race and ethnicity on process and outcomes in health care. In: Unequal Treatment: Confronting Racial and Ethnic Disparities in Health Care. Baltimore, Maryland: Johns Hopkins University; 2003

[94] Zborowski M. Cultural components in response to pain. Journal of Social Issues. 1952;**8**(4):16-30

[95] Zola IK. Culture and symptoms: An analysis of patients' presenting complaints. American Sociological Review. 1966;**31**(5):615-630

[96] Cooper-Patrick L, Gallo JJ, Gonzales JJ, Vu HT, Powe NR, Nelson C, et al. Race, gender, and partnership in the patient-physician relationship. Journal of the American Medical Association. 1999;**282**(6):583-589

[97] Center for Substance Abuse Treatment (US). Improving Cultural Competence. Rockville, MD: Substance Abuse and Mental Health Services Administration (US); 2014 (Treatment Improvement Protocol (TIP) Series, No. 59) 1, Introduction to Cultural Competence. Available from: https://www.ncbi.nlm.nih.gov/books/NBK248431/

[98] DeWalt DA, Malone RM, Bryant ME, Kosnar MC, Corr KE, Rothman RL. A heart failure self-management program for patients of all literacy levels: A randomised, control trial. BMC Health Services Research. 2006;**6**(30):1-10

[99] Rothman R, De Walt D, Malone R, Bryant B, Shintqani A, Crigler B, et al. Influence of patient literacy on the effectiveness of a primary care-based diabetes management program. Journal of the American Medical Association. 2004;**292**(14):1711-1716

Section 2

Managing Patients in the Hospital Setting

Chapter 3

Nutrition and Hospital Mortality, Morbidity and Health Outcomes

Donnette Wright

Abstract

Nutrition has a strong positive linear relationship with hospitalisation, recovery and death. Nutritional status serves as an independent predictor of hospital morbidity and mortality. There is an ensuing academic debate concerning the role and magnitude of nutrition in modifying health outcomes and the strategies that are to be employed to ensure nutritional adequacy. Professional, skill, knowledge and experience are important correlates that may modify patient outcomes, but hospitals continue to be under-resourced even in developed states. It is imperative that current standards, recommendations and policies be examined with the view to aligning the appropriate needs and services to realise positive gains with hospital mortality and morbidity.

Keywords: nutritional adequacy, malnutrition, undernutrition, nutritional support, obesity paradox, hospital mortality

1. Global epidemiology and trends in malnutrition

The incidence of malnutrition has expanded exponentially over the last three decades. At either ends of the nutritional spectrum, malnutrition is concerning to health care professionals and transcends the economic status worldwide, affecting both developed and developing countries. According to the World Health Organization, the incidence of malnutrition is declining among children but remains at critical levels. In 2017, globally there were 151 million children under 5 years of age who were stunted, 51 million children classified as wasted and 38 million children who were overweight. Alternatively, The WHO identifies that global adult undernutrition examined using low body-mass index (BMI) as a proxy has decreased from 13.8% in 1975 to 8.8% in 2014; corresponding levels for women are 14.6 and 9.7%. Conversely, the incidence of malnutrition on the other extreme (overnutrition) was identified as being 1.9 billion among adults (accounting for 38% of the global adult population). Malnutrition has been defined as a health condition where there is an imbalance in the body's supply and usage of energy, protein and other vital nutrients resulting in discernible physiological changes and clinical health outcomes [1]. The epidemiology of malnutrition is difficult to track due to the expansive nature of the definition. Many studies reference malnutrition as undernutrition concerning only weight but the umbrella term also includes conditions of micronutrient deficiencies such as iron, calcium, vitamin A, vitamin D, magnesium, iodine, and vitamin B_{12} which are the leading deficiencies globally. Moreover, overnutrition including overweight and obesity is often not classified as malnutrition, but the concept encompasses these states of nutrition

Burden of disease by cause, World, 2016

Total disease burden, measured in DALYs (Disability-Adjusted Life Years) by sub-categories of disease or injury. DALYs are used to measure total burden of disease - both from years of life lost and years lived with a disability. One DALY equals one lost year of healthy life.

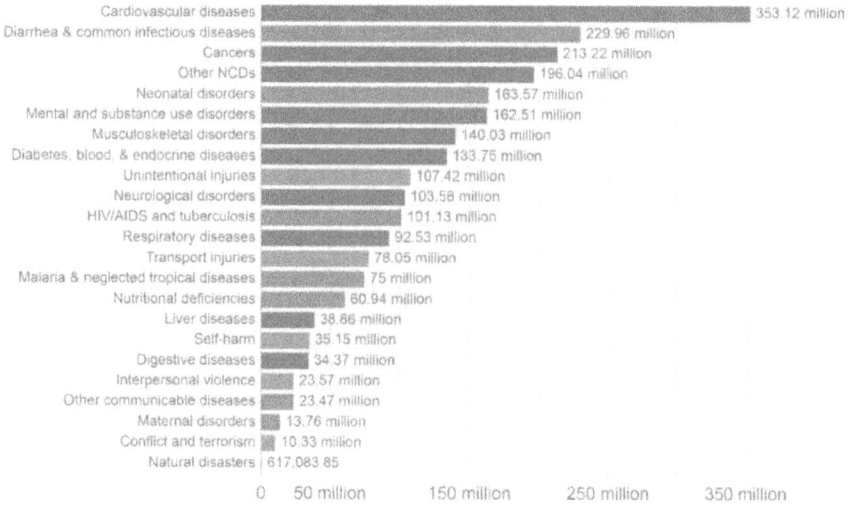

Cardiovascular diseases	353.12 million
Diarrhea & common infectious diseases	229.96 million
Cancers	213.22 million
Other NCDs	196.04 million
Neonatal disorders	163.57 million
Mental and substance use disorders	162.51 million
Musculoskeletal disorders	140.03 million
Diabetes, blood, & endocrine diseases	133.75 million
Unintentional injuries	107.42 million
Neurological disorders	103.58 million
HIV/AIDS and tuberculosis	101.13 million
Respiratory diseases	92.53 million
Transport injuries	78.05 million
Malaria & neglected tropical diseases	75 million
Nutritional deficiencies	60.94 million
Liver diseases	38.86 million
Self-harm	35.15 million
Digestive diseases	34.37 million
Interpersonal violence	23.57 million
Other communicable diseases	23.47 million
Maternal disorders	13.76 million
Conflict and terrorism	10.33 million
Natural disasters	617,083.85

0   50 million   150 million   250 million   350 million

Source: IHME, Global Burden of Disease

CC BY-SA

Figure 1.
The global burden of disease. Source: Ritchie and Roser [2].

and is important in the public health predictions for non-communicable diseases. Nutritional deficiencies are ranked in the top 20 leading worldwide disease and disability burden in 2016, according to the Institute of Health Metrics Evaluation [2], and is a pivotal global concern (see **Figure 1**).

The prevalence of malnutrition in hospitalised adults has been extensively reported in the international literature and varies between 13 and 78% among acute-care patients [3]. Reports pertaining to Latin America describe adult specific values with a much narrower range, with prevalence levels in hospitalised adults totalling 20–50% [4]. The variability in data may be due to tautology of the term, the assessment criteria and variations in institutions. Nevertheless, the impact on health outcomes are consistent across studies.

2. Outcomes of malnutrition

The effects of malnutrition are extensive and include delayed recovery and prolonged hospital stay, increased risk of morbidity and mortality, increased general practitioner visits, and an increased probability of admission to tertiary care facilities [3]. Correspondingly, other literature supports these data and reports that poor nutritional states are associated with increased morbidity and mortality, increased length of hospitalisation, more frequent re-admissions, increased infectious and non-infectious clinical complications and increased healthcare costs [4].

Hospital admissions, duration of hospitalisation and the economic burden of malnutrition have been studied extensively. Contemporary evidence points to a disparity in the length-of-stay (LOS) of adequately-nourished patients when compared with malnourished patients. South African data points to an observation that malnourished patients' LOS approximates 4½ days, which was 43% longer than the stay of the well-nourished patients. Earlier evidence identified an even wider variance between the two states of nutrition, where malnourished patients had demonstrably significantly higher incidence of complications (27.0 vs. 16.8%), increased mortality (12.4 vs. 4.7%), longer LOS (mean of 16.7 vs. 10.1 days) and increased hospital costs [5]. Congruently, Canadian based assessments have also found that malnutrition directly contributes to lengthy hospital stay. After controlling for demographic, socioeconomic, and disease-related factors and treatment, malnutrition at admission was independently associated with prolonged LOS [6]. It was estimated that nutritionally at-risk patients have a fourfold increased cost of hospital care when compared with well-nourished patients in part due to their delay in recovery and the protraction of their hospitalisation. Moreover, in the United Kingdom in 2009, health costs associated with malnutrition was quantified as being at least £13 billion annually [3].

Though undernutrition is a public health issue that undermines the health outcomes of hospitalised patients, malnutrition in the form of overnutrition is also a complex public health challenge with debilitating impact on clinical outcomes and hospitalisations. Worldwide, at least 2.8 million people die each year because of overweight or obesity, and an estimated 35.8 million (2.3%) of global disability adjusted life years (DALYs) are caused by overweight or obesity [7, 8]. Weight related malnutrition is classified by several organisations including CDC, UNICEF [9] and WHO. The World Health Organization's classification is made using weight and height indices and is outlined in **Table 1**.

Current epidemiological data provide concerning evidence of the global expansion of overnutrition. While substantial work has been undertaken to curtail the incidence of undernutrition which has improved over the last decade, there has been a significant increase in the incidence of overnutrition with corresponding increases in the prevalence of non-communicable diseases and poor quality of life.

Classification	BMI (kg/m^2)	
	Principal cut-off points	Additional cut-off points
Underweight	<18.50	<18.50
Severe thinness	<16.00	<16.00
Moderate thinness	16.00–16.99	16.00–16.99
Mild thinness	17.00–18.49	17.00–18.49
Normal range	18.50–24.99	18.50–22.99
		23.00–24.99
Overweight	≥25.00	≥25.00
Pre-obese	25.00–29.99	25.00–27.49
		27.50–29.99
Obese	≥30.00	≥30.00
Obese class I	30.00–34.99	30.00–32.49
		32.50–34.99
Obese class II	35.00–39.99	35.00–37.49
		37.50–39.99
Obese class III	≥40.00	≥40.00

Source: Adapted from WHO (1995, 2000, 2004).

Table 1.
International classification of adult underweight, overweight and obesity using to BMI.

The increase in the rates of obesity and overweight status is not only evident in developing and Agrarian societies but is also featured prominently in industrial societies. **Figure 2** provides a summary of the status of obesity and overweight in WHO regions in 2015 Global Health Observatory data. The WHO makes an even more stark comparison of developing and developing countries, the Organisation suggests that the prevalence of elevated body mass index increases with the income level of countries up to upper middle-income levels. The prevalence of overweight in high income and upper middle-income countries was more than twofold greater than that of low and lower middle-income countries.

Overweight and obesity influence health outcomes and hospitalisation. The prevalence of obesity is high among patients with type 2 diabetes and this may result in the omission of nutritional assessments for these patients [10]. Current evidence also identifies positive health outcomes associated with obesity in specialised admitted patients. European data provide evidence of lower in-hospital mortality and length of ICU stay in overweight and morbidly obese critically ill patients and is consistent with earlier studies that reported better clinical outcomes for critically ill patients with increased BMI [11]. The factors that underpin the physiological benefits of increased BMI in critically ill patients are related to the adequacy of metabolic substrates, the increased capacity for catabolism and increased energy reserves. However, the explanatory factors of improved mortality rates in ICU has not been well examined and many others have been advanced including differences in adipokines and inflammatory mediators, such as leptin and interleukin-10, secreted by fat cells, which are thought to have attenuative inflammatory properties thereby theoretically improving survival during critical illness. Another credible explanation is that persons with higher BMI may have lower severity of illness than their normal BMI counterparts through intangible means [11]. The nutritional status of ICU patients provides an interesting counterpoint to general hospital admissions, however global data on the epidemiology of obesity among patients admitted to ICUs remains limited. Yet, such data are important to understand the possible regional variability of the burden imposed by obesity on outcome and utilisation of healthcare resources. Correspondingly, other European evidence supports this report and identified a concept called the "obesity paradox" where a seemingly negative health condition (overnutrition) is associated with a

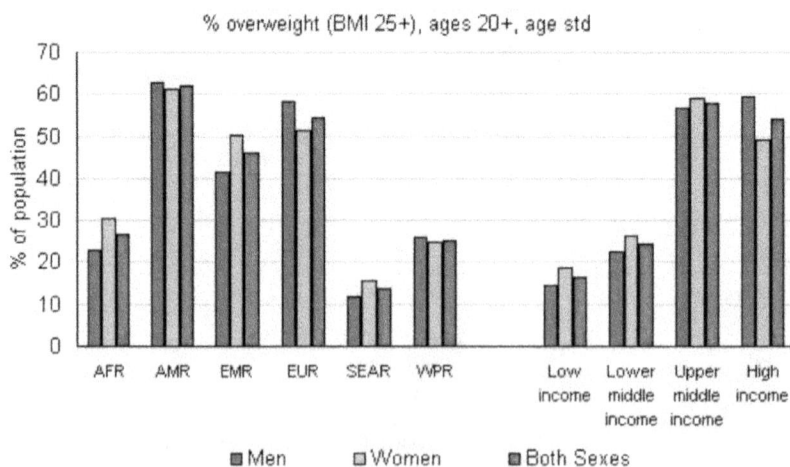

Figure 2.
Global overweight status. Source: [7], concerning WHO regions for Africa, Americas, Eastern Mediterranean, Europe and South East Asia Regions and WHO Western Pacific Region.

positive clinical outcome (reduced hospital length of stay). Shorter hospital stay was reported in populations other than critically ill patients. Parissis et al., [12] found that patients with chronic heart failure, who also had higher BMI had associated lower in-hospital mortality.

Alternatively, and much more common are the negative health outcomes associated with overnutrition. There is a strong positive linear relationship between obesity, overweight and the incidence of non-communicable diseases. There is an analogous increase in the prevalence of comorbidities in tandem with BMI particularly concerning arterial hypertension, diabetes mellitus, and dyslipidaemia. Moreover, current evidence identified that overweight/obese patients represented most of Acute Heart Failure cases, as well as had a higher prevalence of non-cardiovascular comorbidities [12]. Furthermore, North American statistics provide evidence of an inverse near-linear relationship with in-hospital mortality and BMI [12]. Moreover, overnutrition is associated with an increased risk of worsened health status in diabetic patients. The evidence points to poor glycaemic control for obese diabetics when compared to normal weight diabetics [10].

3. Correlates and determinants of malnutrition

The paradigm of malnutrition is considerable, and the concept is linked with many factors. These determinants are usually categorised as clinical and social. **Figure 3** provides a summary of the determinants and correlates of malnutrition.

There are six major physiological factors that are described as influential on malnutrition statuses among people. According to Triantafillidis et al. [14] the six main physical determinants of malnutrition, particularly undernutrition, are:

1. Decrease in oral intake due to primary physiological changes or secondary to health effects

   a. Restrictive diets such as low carb, very low carbohydrate diets (VLCD), low fat, veganism among others

   b. Therapeutic fasting related primarily to presenting health condition such as in gastrointestinal disorders like Crohn's and ulcerative colitis and with bowel prep before gastrointestinal surgeries, or due to diarrhoea, abdominal pain, nausea, and vomiting

   c. Alteration in taste due to drugs, vitamin and mineral deficiencies including in zinc deficiency, and with proinflammatory mediators

   d. Anorexigenous effect of proinflammatory cytokines

2. Gastrointestinal losses which impair energy and nutrient balances

   a. Diarrhoea

   b. Rectorrhagia (rectal bleeding without faeces)/hematochezia (bleeding with stools)

   c. Loss of mucus and electrolytes

   d. Protein-losing enteropathy (disease of the small intestine)

3. Metabolic disorders which interferes with energy balance

   a. Increase in resting energy expenditure due to inflammation, fever, and sepsis

   b. Enhanced fat oxidation

4. Increase in nutritional requirements due to increase substrate requirement for macro and micronutrients with subsequent switch from anabolism to catabolism

   a. Inflammatory states

   b. Increased basal oxidative metabolism—including during fever

   c. Infectious complications-with activated immune response

   d. Postsurgery with substantial tissue repair

5. Drug interactions limiting absorption, digestion and usage of essential micro-nutrients—vitamins, minerals and electrolytes

   a. Corticosteroids and calcium reabsorption

   b. Corticosteroids and protein catabolism—influencing turnover and nitrogen balance

   c. Salazopyrin and folate absorption

   d. Methotrexate and folates

   e. Cholestyramine and fat-soluble vitamins

   f. Antimicrobials esp. cephalosporins and vitamin K; inhibit endogenous metabolism and intestinal absorption

   g. Antisecretors and iron

6. Gastrointestinal or support organ structural dysfunction resulting in poor absorption of nutrients

   a. Reduction of the absorptive surface due to intestinal resection and enteric fistulas and high output fistulas

   b. Blind loops and bacterial overgrowth

   c. Poor absorption of bile salts in ileitis or resection

   d. Mucosal inflammation and inflammatory diseases [14]

Alternately, the determinants of overnutrition are fewer and varies widely from those resulting in undernutrition, however the concept of energy and food intake is consistent across malnutrition categories. There are definitive proponents of obesity

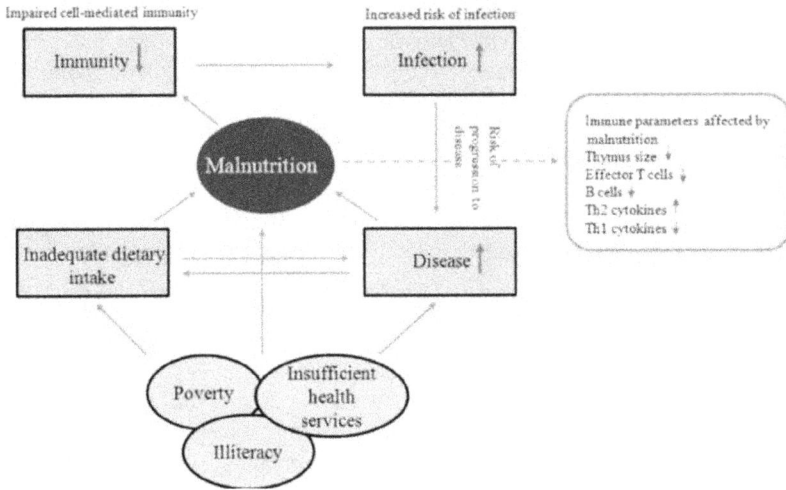

Figure 3.
Factors influencing malnutrition. Source: Bapat et al. [13], p. 2.

development. It is documented that increased consumption of energy dense foods which are correspondingly poor in micronutrients, greater than physiologic demand will lead to weight accumulation, shifting the beam of the pendulum from balance to excess [10]. North American data identifies biological, behavioural and social contributors of obesity, insomuch as Lifshitz and Lifshitz [15] proposes that the causes of obesity are multifactorial, they include:

1. A genetic predisposition

2. Hormonal activity

3. Health status and disease burden

4. An environmental susceptibility to gain weight

5. Increased energy intake

6. Reduced energy expenditures

7. Structural environmental changes creating an obesogenic environment

8. Abundance of high-caloric density, low-quality food

9. Food selection/preparation

10. National and international food policies

The factors increasing the risk of malnutrition exist for malnourished states central to as well as external to hospitalisation. Though the factors outlined hitherto contributes significantly to hospital-based malnutrition, the unique concept of hospitalisations worsens the risk and the incidence of malnutrition. In secondary care facilities malnutrition, and more frequently undernutrition, develops as a result of insufficient energy and nutrient intake, impaired digestion/absorption/

utilisation or loss of nutrients due to illness or trauma through wounds, fistulas, or excreta as well increased metabolic demands during illness, recovery, and physiological response [4]. There remains no consensus on the definition of malnutrition, especially undernutrition, with a profusion of criteria possibly explaining some of the inconsistencies in the prevalence rates reported in the literature. Generally, unintentional weight loss >5% in a short period of time (over 3–6 months) and decreased food intake are among the definitive parameters of undernutrition [4]. Consistent with the challenges in defining malnutrition, so too is there challenge in delineating all the factors that correlate with malnutrition, particularly undernutrition.

Supportive evidence precedes these assertions and describe the causes of "disease-related malnutrition" as being inclusive of insufficient food/nutrient intake, impaired nutrient digestion and absorption and increased requirements for nutrients with increased losses (e.g., from wounds, malabsorption) and catabolism [1]. While other evidence points to a strong social link, where nutritional status at hospital admission is said to be compounded by primary malnutrition mainly reflecting poor socioeconomic conditions, and secondary malnutrition usually influenced by the impact of degenerative, terminal and chronic diseases [16].

Acute malnutrition takes place in a few weeks to months, it primarily affects lean body stores and is usually managed effectively to prevent permanent impact, especially in children. It occurs in a range of instances including during emergencies, seasonally and endemically [17]. These situations usually contribute to undernutrition through severe restrictions to nutrient and energy supply. In the former case, hospital-based emergencies may result in medium term therapeutic fasts, while in countries which rely heavily on agriculture and have variable weather pattern, food security may be critically impacted creating a unique form of dietary restriction. In undernutrition, there is a greater risk of death which is related not only to the infection but also to the loss of muscle mass with concordant limits to immunity and primary metabolic functions. Fat stores, which are used up in cases of undernutrition without infection, may also play a role in survival and regulate bone linear growth [17].

4. At risk groups

In as much as malnutrition is debilitating and associated with severe health outcomes, there are vulnerable groups for which malnutrition, particularly undernutrition, is more likely to affect and by extension more probable to result in death. The literature suggest that malnutrition is a problem in many different disease groups, including cancer (5–80%), neurology (4–66%), surgical/critical illness (0–100%), respiratory disease (5–60%), gastrointestinal and liver disease (3–100%), HIV/AIDS (8–98%) and renal disease (10–72%) [1]. Over a similar period in Cuba the rates of undernutrition were alarming 41.2% were classified as undernourished and 11.1% of patients were considered severely undernourished. Malnutrition rates increased progressively with prolonged length of stay [18]. Current evidence highlights that patients who are hospitalised are at risk of developing iatrogenic malnutrition or hospital-based malnutrition due to several reasons. Patients admitted in hospitals, for instance after an acute exacerbation of a chronic condition, are at high risk of developing disease-related malnutrition (DRM) a consequence of loss of appetite, poor nutritional intake, and disease-related catabolism and in severe instances cachexia [19]. In addition to the clinical conditions that may predispose patients to malnutrition, age and gender are also factors which create additional risk. Children and infants with limited physiological and nutritional reserves, pregnant women who must physically meet her needs and that of a growing foetus as well as the elderly are numbered among the vulnerable, nutritionally at-risk group. Hospitalised elderly patients are particularly vulnerable to develop DRM because of poor nutritional antecedents including decreased fat free mass and impaired protein, energy, and fluid intake [19]. Consequently, care must be taken to screen, assess, manage and follow up patients who are at-risk of malnutrition in an effort to reduce the associated risk of mortality and morbidity across differing health conditions/disease states and the lifecycle [20].

5. Malnutrition across the lifespan

Negative health outcomes resulting from poor nutrition is pervasive across all life stages and impacts individuals differently in each group due to physiological and developmental differences among groups. Consequently, health care professionals must be keen to ensure that the unique characteristics and risks in each group are evaluated. Therefore, international organisations such as PAHO, WHO and CDC have instituted concerted efforts, but the rates and impact of childhood malnutrition continues to be extensive. Childhood is characterized by a period of dependence, rapid growth and limited nutritional reserves accordingly, parental neglect, limited knowledge and socioeconomic capacity may negatively influence nutritional adequacy. Globally childhood malnutrition continues to be a public health problem with alarming statistics in 2015, out of the 1.5 million children who died, nearly half (45%) of these deaths resulted from malnutrition or its correlates [21]. In the Latin America and the Caribbean, the rates are more concerning with infant mortality rate being 11 per 1000 live births in Barbados [22]. Furthermore, infants and children exposed earlier and more sustainably to poor states of nutrition have a greater probability of experiencing more severe and chronic health outcomes as a result. In utero as well as cohort studies of the Latin Americas and the Caribbean and European societies suggest that foetus exposed to poor maternal nutrition, and children 0–6 months old exposed to poor nutritional profiles are more likely to be hospitalised, exhibit mental disorders such as personality and schizoid disorders and have chronic diseases including hypertension and diabetes [22, 23]. Moreover, European evidence points to greater episodes of diarrhoea, vomiting, poor recovery, longer hospital stays and greater health care costs in admitted children with body mass indices less than two standard deviations in children compared to healthy controls [24]. Nevertheless, the morbidity associated with nutritional inadequacies in children can be attenuated with early and appropriate nutritional interventions. Studies concerning the Caribbean and West African population have shown that the rate of hospitalisation and mental illness associated with poor childhood nutrition declined with nutritional supplementation in both Barbados and Mauritius [23].

Similar to the physiological impact in infancy and childhood, pregnancy and lactation create nutritional vulnerabilities for the foetus and the mother. The additional metabolic demands, nutritional requirements of the foetus and the capacity to support the organ changes coupled with emotional and physiological factors limiting dietary intake increase the risk of nutritional inadequacy in pregnancy. Current evidence suggests that it increases the risk of morbidity and mortality for both the mother and the unborn child. In Latin America, there are reports of a lack of specialised tool to examine maternal nutritional states as well as a lack of protocols to guide nutritional support and intervention [21]. In pregnancy, poor maternal weight gain, low haemoglobin levels, and impaired fasting plasma glucose levels, as well as poor maternal dietary intake and physical inactivity are important predictors of infant mortality, maternal mortality, low birth weight and poor infant growth and development [21]. The authors suggest that assessment, screening, follow-up and maternal care are important modulators of these outcomes.

For adolescents, the portion of the lifecycle is characterized by rapid growth and organ development, greater autonomy and independence, access to media and dietary advice. Contingent on the adolescent's support and capacity to negotiate these changes he may be at risk of developing micronutrient deficiencies such as iron and calcium, or experience macronutrient imbalances associated with obesity and wasting as well as eating disorders such as anorexia nervosa and bulimia [25]. Growth should be monitored at regular intervals throughout childhood and adolescence and should also be measured every time an adolescent visits a healthcare facility for preventive, acute, or chronic care. In children ages 2–20 years several nutritional and developmental indices should be measured as a standard procedure to identify and treat potential nutritional risks and disorders including standing height-for-age, weight-for-age, and body mass index (BMI)-for-age [26].

While adolescence malnutrition is plagued with equal risks of acute and chronic outcomes, in adulthood the risks associated with nutritional imbalances have greater links to chronic illnesses such as cardiovascular and endocrine disorders. These disorders worsen morbidity risk in nutritionally unhealthy adults through poorer quality of life and longer periods of disability adjusted life years (DALY) mainly as a result of the contribution of overweight and obesity. Similarly, underweight, using mid upper arm circumference as a proxy for assessment, has shown strong negative correlations with in-hospital mortality in adults. It accounted for a nearly (3.8) fourfold increased risk of in-hospital mortality when compared with healthy controls [27]. Other evidence points however to a protective effect of obesity on in-hospital mortality in adults where odds of death was 0.9 and 0.7 in overweight and obese patients compared to normal weight adult counterparts. Other evidence however confirmed the findings of Asiimwe [27] inasmuch as it reports that the odds of dying were higher in hospitalised undernourished adult patients [28].

Nutritional health maintenance and its sequelae of outcomes are similarly perplexing in the elderly. They have a double burden of increased micronutrient requirements such as iron, calcium, and phosphorus with a discordant reduction in the requirement for macronutrients. In the face of this conundrum, the health care provider must be careful of the nutritional prescriptions to balance macronutrient requirements to attenuate chronic disease risk as well as to maintain adequate micronutrient requirements to prevent and manage important metabolic changes associated with the physiological features of aging. Furthermore, the older adult is described as nutritionally vulnerable because he has reduced physical reserve that restricts the ability to mount a vigorous recovery when there is an acute health threat or stressor [29]. In developing as well as developed countries malnutrition is identified as an independent predictor of mortality. The mortality rate in malnourished elderly Brazilians aged between 60 and 69 years was 3.34 deaths per 1000 inhabitants, and among those aging 70 years and older, 11 deaths per 1000 inhabitants [30]. The factors contributing to the elderly's nutritional vulnerability include multiple medical conditions, and polypharmacy, physiological changes affecting intake and absorption including xerostomia, anorexia of aging and achlorhydria, obesity, and limited socioeconomic resources. Conversely, having adequate muscle mass, replete micronutrient stores, healthy dietary practices and adequate social support are protective factors against nutritional inadequacy in the elderly population [29]. Consistent across all life stages is the risk of nutritional ill health, unique to each segment of the cycle is a physiological and development paradigm that creates a distinctive risk for the individual. Critical to the successful negotiation of the life stage is the public health role that providers play, they must be equipped to screen, assess, diagnose, and prescribe appropriate individualised plans and evaluate nutritional outcomes. It is important therefore for the health care provider to be conversant regarding the procedures for managing both elements of the spectrum of malnutrition.

6. Management of malnutrition

Comparable with the debate concerning the criteria for defining undernutrition, there continues to be a rigorous academic discourse surrounding the management of undernutrition.

Though the debate is still raging, institutes such as BAPEN, ASPEN and ESPEN and health professionals have advanced nutritional prescriptions linked to the energy, amino acid and electrolyte needs. Protein and energy supply in undernourished patients contribute to supporting metabolic reactions, providing substrates for immune functions and expansion of lean body reserves, while electrolytes and major minerals such as iron, sodium, phosphorus and potassium are essential for electrical and neuronal conductivity and several metabolic homeostatic reactions. Energy and protein recommendations are usually the most varied elements of the debate, nevertheless contemporary and classical evidence converges on the general recommendations for nutritional support of undernourished clients. These patients should be prescribed a diet based on the following allowances: protein, 1.1–1.5 g/kg; calories, 30–35 kcal/kg; sodium, 87–120 mEq/day; potassium, 1.1–1.5 mEq/kg; phosphorus, <17 mg/kg. Additional nutritional supports in the form of high-protein or high-protein and high-calorie supplements were also provided to individual patients whose weight was <80% of their habitual body weight, if they had more than 3 kg (5–7 lb) of weight loss in a month, and/or their serum albumin was <3.5 g/dl [31, 32]. Despite the benefits that can be accrued from nutritional support, the problem is still evident in the Low and Middle-Income countries of the Latin Americas. In eight Latin American countries (Argentina, Brazil, Chile, Colombia, Ecuador, Mexico, Panama, and Peru), malnutrition was found to be prevalent among hospitalised patients and caloric intake failed to meet targeted energy delivery in 40% of hospitalised adults receiving nutrition therapy. The evidence suggested that supplemental administration of parenteral and enteral nutrition was associated with improved energy and protein delivery and reduced mortality levels [33].

For children, malnutrition-especially undernutrition may be more incestuous and accompanied by infectious diseases, worm and helminth infections and involve both macro and micronutrient deficiencies. Current evidence outlines that childhood malnutrition is a significant contributor to mortality rates of children under five. The risk of death may be attenuated by energy supply dependent on calorimetric determinants and earlier antibiotic therapy [34].

7. Nutritional screening, assessment and evaluation

To effectively manage undernutrition, patients' nutritional status must be determined, and the nutritional prescription individualised based on their needs. Screening and assessment are the procedures necessary for the classification of client's nutritional status. Furthermore, nutritional risk screening is an important modulator of mortality and morbidity risk particularly in hospitalised surgical patients [35]. Current research supports this finding, as nutritional screening is described as one of the most critical initial steps in nutritional management. Many health care professional groups (ASPEN, BAPEN and ESPEN) currently recommend nutritional screening of acute care patients, either before elective admissions or within 24–48 h after emergency admissions. It is imperative to identify and classify malnourished patients promptly to prevent or counter the associated negative health outcomes. Currently, physicians and nurses assess patients on admission to hospital, and it has been suggested that they are in an ideal position to screen patients for malnutrition [3]. Moreover, clinicians suggest that nutritional status evaluation include clinical and biochemical assessments. Standard biochemical assessments should include basic serum electrolyte tests as well as serum albumin and prealbumin levels which are direct markers of lean body mass. For several authors, serum albumin level is the best prognostic indicator of nutritional status because of its ability to detect protein-energy malnutrition, which may not be accompanied by declines in body mass index and body weight or may be sub-clinical especially in the acute phases. Additionally, serum albumin level was identified a better predictor of some types of morbidity, particularly sepsis and major infections, than other types [36].

Effective nutritional management strategies include: appropriate weighing practices; documentation of weight fluctuations; monitoring of biochemical parameters and food intake; and clear malnutrition identification criteria through nutritional screening. Using nutritional experts and multidisciplinary nutritional teams is also recommended to help combat malnutrition [3].

Furthermore, there abounds a plethora of algorithms that outlines effective nutritional management procedures inclusive of screening, assessment and intervention guidelines. There are disease specific algorithms as well as population specific protocols available including guidelines from ASPEN as outlined in **Figure 4**.

Algorithms such as the one advanced by ASPEN are available and supported by hospital protocols but there remains low levels of nutritional screening and assessment particularly in resource restricted low-income countries such as Latin America and the Caribbean, the rates are troubling. In a study of 14 countries, only two were found to have national policies regarding best practices for nutrition therapy in hospitals or long-term care facilities and this data was associated with only 9% of patients who required parenteral or enteral nutrition receiving the treatment [4].

In children, several indices have been identified by health authorities including the WHO as being suitable in identifying malnutrition and its risk. Current evidence points to mid-upper-arm circumference (MUAC) providing better estimates of childhood mortality when compared with weight-for-height. Weight-for-height is unstable and variable in acute conditions affecting body water. It is

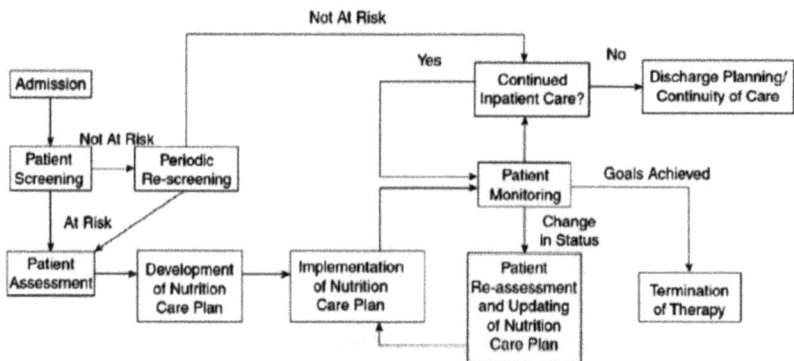

Figure 4.
Nutrition care algorithm. Source: [37], p. 17.

more sensitive to dehydration, such as in the case of diarrhoea, where dehydration causes weight loss with little impact on lean body mass [17], therefore MUAC which is more robust against these changes, is recommended as a more stable measure of nutritional status and risk.

8. Professional and nutrition care

Consistent with the need for nutritional screening, assessment and evaluation, is the poignant value of hospitals and primary as well as tertiary care facilities being staffed with professionals knowledgeable, skilled and resourced to deliver adequate nutritional support. In stark contrast to this recommendation is the reality of the characteristics of human resources that people these institutions. In some studies, provider knowledge, understanding and data usage was identified as a barrier to optimal nutritional support [38]. In Swedish settings, limited access to nutrition related education as well as availability of training programmes were identified as having negative effects on nutritional support and management [39]. Furthermore, there is low nutrition related health literacy among health care professionals partly attributable to a weak "nutritional culture" correspondent with inadequate academic training and preparation of health care professionals [40]. This partly due to limits in the nutritional education and training afforded to health care providers.

> *"The quantity of formalized nutrition education is shrinking in the curricula of health professions, such as physicians, nurses, dietitians, and pharmacists. The current nutrition education being taught in U.S. schools of healthcare professionals does not appropriately prepare students for identification of patients at nutrition risk or management of undernourished hospitalized patients with specialized nutrition therapies...."* ([41] p. 218).

While health care workers recognised the value of nutritional screening and assessment, deficiencies in their knowledge and skill limit the benefits that could be accrued from early and consistent nutritional evaluation. Coupled with individual level limitations there are also policy level challenges as well as institutional and nationally challenges in some respects [39]. In the Latin America, the culture, value, and significance of nutritional support in health care are limited even as the prevalence of malnutrition and its outcomes rise. The increased rates of community and hospital malnutrition and its morbidity and mortality risks in Latin America occur alongside a limitation in the awareness levels of providers concerning the management of disease-related malnutrition [42]. It however, represents an opportunity to improve nutrition care by increasing education and training. Healthcare administrators, clinical leaders and educators, and clinicians must first recognise the significance of nutrition to health care and then must be knowledgeable in order to realise the benefits of nutritional support in hospitals.

Though there are inconsistencies in the proponents' views on the diagnosis and treatment of malnutrition there is consensus on the need for treatment and the value of nutritional support to health care outcomes. Current guidelines published by the European Society for Clinical Nutrition and Metabolism (ESPEN) provide primarily recommendations for nutritional therapy specific to organ/system dysfunctions and medical specialty [19]. However, large developed and developing countries fail to institute these recommendations in the abundance and the absence of adequate resources. Knowledge, experience, self-confidence, and self-efficacy may be the intangible factors constraining the implementation of these guidelines. Current evidence points to their impact on negative clinical and health outcomes including worsening risk of mortality and morbidity as a consequence of under-treatment of vulnerable hospitalised patients.

Significantly, developed and emerging societies are plagued with malnutrition and its consequences as well as institutional and provider level incompetencies to manage the spiralling problem. The burden is more severe in resource restricted countries. To attenuate the negative effects of malnutrition developing countries should employ the following strategies:

1. Evaluate, adopt and customise appropriate nutritional management algorithms to guide health care practitioners

2. Institute appropriate national and institutional policies to guide and support the use of nutritional treatment protocols

3. Assess the training and educational needs of the health care teams

4. Organise regular and contemporary education/training procedures and updates for all members of the health care team

5. Engender a culture of nutritional significance and value to health care development and recovery

6. Reinforce nutritional evaluation and follow-up during and post hospitalisation

7. Adopt international primary and public health strategies to minimize primary malnutrition risk

8. Support the documentation of unique nutritional support procedures and the statistics concerning nutritional management

9. Conclusion

The global incidence of malnutrition is significant. Nutritional inadequacies directly impact hospital morbidity and mortality rates, worsening death for the most parts and to a lesser extent obesity has been linked to a protective effect. The condition severely diminishes quality of life for individuals of all ages. Health care providers through their capacity and responsibility to screen, assess and intervene serve as critical modulators of malnutrition outcomes. Nevertheless, their attenuative capacity is severely restricted through limited nutrition health related culture, training, education and resource limitations. Notwithstanding the significant challenges, countries and health care institutions must recognise the role nutrition plays in morbidity and mortality and institute effective action, including training and education, as well as policy and resource provision in order to stymie the negative impact of nutrition on morbidity and mortality.

Author details

Donnette Wright
The UWI School of Nursing, Mona, University of the West Indies, Jamaica,
West Indies

*Address all correspondence to: donnette.wright02@uwimona.edu.jm

IntechOpen

References

[1] Meier R, Stratton R. Basic concepts in nutrition: Epidemiology of malnutrition. European e-Journal of Clinical Nutrition and Metabolism. 2008;**3**(4):e167-e170

[2] Ritchie H, Roser M. Micronutrient Deficiency. 2018. Published online at OurWorldInData.org. Retrieved from: https://ourworldindata.org/micronutrient-deficiency

[3] van Tonder E, Gardner L, Cressey S, Tydeman-Edwards R, Gerber K. Adult malnutrition: Prevalence and use of nutrition-related quality indicators in South African public-sector hospitals. South African Journal of Clinical Nutrition. 2017;**32**(1):1-7

[4] Correia MIT, Perman MI, Waitzberg DL. Hospital malnutrition in Latin America: A systematic review. Clinical Nutrition. 2017;**36**(4):958-967

[5] Correia MIT, Waitzberg DL. The impact of malnutrition on morbidity, mortality, length of hospital stay and costs evaluated through a multivariate model analysis. Clinical Nutrition. 2003;**22**(3):235-239

[6] Allard JP, Keller H, Jeejeebhoy KN, Laporte M, Duerksen DR, Gramlich L, et al. Malnutrition at hospital admission—Contributors and effect on length of stay: A prospective cohort study from the Canadian Malnutrition Task Force. Journal of Parenteral and Enteral Nutrition. 2016;**40**(4):487-497

[7] World Health Organization. Global Health Observatory (GHO) Data. 2016. Child Mortality and Causes of Death. Geneva: WHO; 2016

[8] WHO, UNICEF, Mathers C. Global strategy for women's, children's and adolescents' health (2016-2030). Organization. 2017;**2016**(9)

[9] UNICEF/WHO/World Bank Group. Joint child malnutrition estimates: Key findings of the 2017 edition. 2017. Retrieved from: http://www.who.int/news-room/commentaries/detail/double-duty-actions-for-ending-malnutrition-within-a-decade

[10] Yildirim ZG, Uzunlulu M, Caklili OT, Mutlu HH, Oguz A. Malnutrition rate among hospitalized patients with type 2 diabetes mellitus. Progress in Nutrition. 2018;**20**(2):183-188

[11] Sakr Y, Alhussami I, Nanchal R, Wunderink RG, Pellis T, Wittebole X, et al. Being overweight is associated with greater survival in ICU patients: Results from the intensive care over nations audit. Critical Care Medicine. 2015;**43**(12):2623-2632

[12] Parissis J, Farmakis D, Kadoglou N, Ikonomidis I, Fountoulaki E, Hatziagelaki E, et al. Body mass index in acute heart failure: Association with clinical profile, therapeutic management and in-hospital outcome. European Journal of Heart Failure. 2016;**18**(3):298-305

[13] Bapat PR, Satav AR, Husain AA, Shekhawat SD, Kawle AP, Chu JJ, et al. Differential levels of alpha-2-macroglobulin, haptoglobin and sero-transferrin as adjunct markers for TB diagnosis and disease progression in the malnourished tribal population of Melghat, India. PLoS One. 2015;**10**(8):e0133928

[14] Triantafillidis JK, Vagianos C, Papalois AE. The role of enteral nutrition in patients with inflammatory bowel disease: Current aspects. BioMed Research International. 2015;**2015**:1-13

[15] Lifshitz F, Lifshitz JZ. Globesity: The root causes of the obesity epidemic in the USA and now worldwide. Pediatric Endocrinology Reviews: PER. 2014;**12**(1):17-34

[16] Goiburu ME, Jure Goiburu MM, Bianco H, Ruiz Díaz J, Alderete F, Palacios MC, et al. The impact of malnutrition on morbidity, mortality and length of hospital stay in trauma patients. Nutrición Hospitalaria. 2006;**21**(5):604-610

[17] de Pee S, Grais R, Fenn B, Brown R, Briend A, Frize J, et al. Prevention of acute malnutrition: Distribution of special nutritious foods and cash, and addressing underlying causes—What to recommend when, where, for whom, and how. Food and Nutrition Bulletin. 2015;**36**(1_suppl1):S24-S29

[18] Penié JB, Cuban Group for the Study of Hospital Malnutrition. State of malnutrition in Cuban hospitals. Nutrition. 2005;**21**(4):487-497

[19] Bounoure L, Gomes F, Stanga Z, Keller U, Meier R, Ballmer P, et al. Detection and treatment of medical inpatients with or at-risk of malnutrition: Suggested procedures based on validated guidelines. Nutrition. 2016;**32**(7-8):790-798

[20] Cederholm T, Bosaeus I, Barazzoni R, Bauer J, Van Gossum A, Klek S, et al. Diagnostic criteria for malnutrition— An ESPEN consensus statement. Clinical Nutrition. 2015;**34**(3):335-340

[21] LaMontagne M, Miller B, Falcone T. Development and implementation of a nutritional-risk screening procedure for pregnant mothers in a Honduran community hospital system. 2017;**587**: 1-21

[22] Hock RS, Bryce CP, Waber DP, McCuskee S, Fitzmaurice GM, Henderson DC, et al. Relationship between infant malnutrition and childhood maltreatment in a Barbados lifespan cohort. Vulnerable Children and Youth Studies. 2017;**12**(4):304-316

[23] Hock RS, Bryce CP, Fischer L, First MB, Fitzmaurice GM, Costa

PT, et al. Childhood malnutrition and maltreatment are linked with personality disorder symptoms in adulthood: Results from a Barbados lifespan cohort. Psychiatry Research. 2018;**269**:301-308

[24] Hecht C, Weber M, Grote V, Daskalou E, Dell'Era L, Flynn D, et al. Disease associated malnutrition correlates with length of hospital stay in children. Clinical Nutrition. 2015;**34**(1):53-59

[25] Garber AK, Machen VI, Park CC, Peebles R. Changing approaches to refeeding malnourished patients with eating disorders: Results of an International Survey. Journal of Adolescent Health. 2018;**62**(2):S100

[26] Becker P, Carney LN, Corkins MR, Monczka J, Smith E, Smith SE, et al. Consensus statement of the Academy of Nutrition and Dietetics/American Society for Parenteral and Enteral Nutrition: Indicators recommended for the identification and documentation of pediatric malnutrition (undernutrition). Nutrition in Clinical Practice. 2015;**30**(1):147-161

[27] Asiimwe SB. Simplifications of the mini nutritional assessment short-form are predictive of mortality among hospitalized young and middle-aged adults. Nutrition. 2016;**32**(1):95-100

[28] Cereda E, Klersy C, Hiesmayr M, Schindler K, Singer P, Laviano A, et al. Body mass index, age and in-hospital mortality: The Nutrition Day multinational survey. Clinical Nutrition. 2017;**36**(3):839-847

[29] Starr KNP, McDonald SR, Bales CW. Nutritional vulnerability in older adults: A continuum of concerns. Current Nutrition Reports. 2015;**4**(2):176-184

[30] Damião R, Santos ÁDS, Matijasevich A, Menezes PR. Factors

associated with risk of malnutrition in the elderly in south-eastern Brazil. Revista Brasileira de Epidemiologia. 2017;**20**:598-610

[31] Fleischmann E, Teal N, Dudley J, May W, Bower JD, Salahudeen AK. Influence of excess weight on mortality and hospital stay in 1346 hemodialysis patients. Kidney International. 1999;**55**(4):1560-1567

[32] Park J, Ahmadi SF, Streja E, Molnar MZ, Flegal KM, Gillen D, et al. Obesity paradox in end-stage kidney disease patients. Progress in Cardiovascular Diseases. 2014;**56**(4):415-425

[33] Vallejo KP, Martínez CM, Adames AAM, Fuchs-Tarlovsky V, Nogales GCC, Paz RER, et al. Current clinical nutrition practices in critically ill patients in Latin America: A multinational observational study. Critical Care. 2017;**21**(1):227

[34] Trehan I, Goldbach HS, LaGrone LN, Meuli GJ, Wang RJ, Maleta KM, et al. Research article (New England Journal of Medicine) antibiotics as part of the management of severe acute malnutrition. Malawi Medical Journal. 2016;**28**(3):123-130

[35] Schwegler I, Von Holzen A, Gutzwiller JP, Schlumpf R, Mühlebach S, Stanga Z. Nutritional risk is a clinical predictor of postoperative mortality and morbidity in surgery for colorectal cancer. British Journal of Surgery. 2010;**97**(1):92-97

[36] Alves A, Panis Y, Mathieu P, Mantion G, Kwiatkowski F, Slim K. Postoperative mortality and morbidity in French patients undergoing colorectal surgery: Results of a prospective multicenter study. Archives of Surgery. 2005;**140**(3):278-283

[37] Mueller C, Compher C, Ellen DM, American Society for Parenteral and Enteral Nutrition (ASPEN) Board of Directors. ASPEN clinical guidelines: Nutrition screening, assessment, and intervention in adults. Journal of Parenteral and Enteral Nutrition. 2011;**35**(1):16-24

[38] Martin L, de van der Schueren MA, Blauwhoff-Buskermolen S, Baracos V, Gramlich L. Identifying the barriers and enablers to nutrition care in head and neck and esophageal cancers: An international qualitative study. Journal of Parenteral and Enteral Nutrition. 2016;**40**(3):355-366

[39] Duerksen DR, Keller HH, Vesnaver E, Laporte M, Jeejeebhoy K, Payette H, et al. Nurses' perceptions regarding the prevalence, detection, and causes of malnutrition in Canadian hospitals: Results of a Canadian Malnutrition Task Force Survey. Journal of Parenteral and Enteral Nutrition. 2016;**40**(1):100-106

[40] Donini LM, Leonardi F, Rondanelli M, Banderali G, Battino M, Bertoli E, et al. The domains of human nutrition: The importance of nutrition education in academia and medical schools. Frontiers in Nutrition. 2017;**4**:2

[41] Sacks GS. The shrinking of formalized nutrition education in health professions curricula and postgraduate training. Journal of Parenteral and Enteral Nutrition. 2017;**41**(2):217-225

[42] Correia MI, Hegazi RA, Diaz-Pizarro Graf JI, Gomez-Morales G, Fuentes Gutiérrez C, Goldin MF, et al. Addressing disease-related malnutrition in healthcare: A Latin American perspective. Journal of Parenteral and Enteral Nutrition. 2016;**40**(3):319-325

Chapter 4

Improving the Quality of Care in Surgery: The Role of Guidelines, Protocols, Checklist and the Multidisciplinary Team

Joseph Martin Plummer, Mark S. Newnham and Timothy Henry

Abstract

Today's surgical environment is a complex multifaceted one that has eroded the traditional doctor patient relationship. Increasingly a discerning public expects surgery to be efficiently performed and be free of complications. Decisions about choosing a doctor are now data driven and the health system must adapt accordingly in order to attract patients. The streamlining of the patient: treatment: outcome continuum can be made better with the use of various standard operating procedures such as the use of guidelines, protocols and checklists with a multidisciplinary team where all stakeholders are actively engaged. This is especially important in developing countries for the potential savings in lives and finances. Still the need for individualization and good clinical judgment remains. The basis of all our decisions however must be evidence-based, and once applied in the best interest of the patient will benefit health care systems. There is good evidence that this is the case, and the only limitation currently is the lack of more widespread implementation.

Keywords: quality of surgery, guidelines, checklists and protocols, multidisciplinary teams

1. Introduction

Medical knowledge is increasing at an exponential pace and as such standard of care applicable a decade ago may not necessarily apply today, depending on the condition and the level of evidence supporting the change. Patients now have access to a wide range of information, proportionate on their resources, motivation and level of education. In fact they can be seen no longer as 'patients' but 'clients' who are consumers and shoppers of care. As such they expect that their doctors will be professional, compassionate and with up-to-date knowledge and skills, providing at least a basic standard of care that *guarantees* a good outcome. The duty of a certain standard is owed to the public by the doctors, nurses, administrators, and all other members of the health team irrespective of the patient's resources, social class or religion.

Oftentimes there is a gap in new medical knowledge and its translation to clinical practice, and on average this can take up to a decade [1, 2]. The consequences of these evidence-to-practice gaps are potentially significant, with risk of mortality, morbidity and significant healthcare and financial impact. Importantly, once there is a concerted effort to improve quality in clinical care, gradually over time we will see improved results [3, 4] across the spectrum of quality outcomes. For example there is evidence that cancer outcome can be improved by up to 30% with optimum application of best evidence with a 10% reduction in cancer mortality if the evidence for best practice was used.

Confronted with overwhelming evidence that substantial harm was being done to the public due to inadequate patient safety and the failure to practice using the best currently available evidence, the World Health Assembly (WHA) mandated the WHO to take a lead in setting global norms and standards and supporting countries in preparing patient safety policies and practices [5]. In 2008 the WHO choose the 'safety of surgical care' for its second Global Patient Safety Challenge. This Safe Surgery Saves Lives Program brought together surgeons, gynecologists, anesthetists, ward and theater nurses, operating theater managers, patient advocates, infection control experts and biomedical engineers to identify opportunities to improve the safety of surgical patients [6]. The groups were tasked with considering four pillars for improved outcome: infection prevention, anesthetic safety, teamwork and communication and measurement of surgical capacity and outcomes. It has been a decade since the launch of this mandate and although the measures identified were not new, they certainly brought into focus the importance of clinical practice guidelines, checklists and protocols as tools available to improve the quality of surgical care. Increasingly more recently especially with the importance of a multimodal approach to the treatment of cancers, an additional area of focus to improve the quality of surgical care is the role of multidisciplinary rounds.

The process for the successful systems improvement was divided into three stages: teaching, which has a widely variable performance rate; mandates/regulations, which results in modest level of performance improvement; and systemization including data feedback loops, coaching, and checklists, which result in high reliability [7]. Once implemented, this improvement is noticeable both at 'well-performing' hospitals and 'worse-performing' hospitals [8] and would have a substantial impact in achieving more from the limited spending allocated annually in the national budget to healthcare. This is because meaningful implementation of these safety measures occurs when there is a shift in the mindset of the surgeon from solo practitioners (autonomous cowboys) to a team-based or 'pit crew' approach. Dr. Gawande [7] noted that this change in the operating room involves humility, discipline, and teamwork. He emphasized three critical pause points for surgery as identified by the checklist: before the induction of anesthesia, before the incision in the skin, and before the patient leaves the operating room (OR). Whereas the purpose of the checklist was to help the OR team remember important details that may be missed during an operation, it certainly encourages teamwork and communication.

2. The scope of the problem

Surgical care is essential in improving population health. It is estimated that there is one operation performed annually for every 25 human beings alive [9]. With this volume there is a great potential source for a public health crisis. Globally perioperative mortality has declined significantly over the past 50 years, with the greatest decline in developed countries. It is in developing countries where avoidable surgical complications disproportionately account for a large proportion of preventable medical injuries and deaths globally [10]. A surgical complication is any undesirable, unintended and direct result of an operation affecting the patient that would not have occurred had the operation gone well as could reasonably be hoped [11]. Whereas complications of medical care may occur as a consequence of both the illness and the treatment, in general its regarded as 'a complication' when it was not caused by the underlying disease [12]. This 'complication' is perhaps better labeled 'an adverse event' which is defined as an unintended injury caused by medical management rather than by the underlying disease or condition of the patient [13]. In developed countries up to 17% of all inpatient surgeries will have a major complication [14]. Nearly 30% of all adverse events were as a result of negligence, and these events were much higher in the elderly. Often complications occur as a result of errors of commission or acts of omission. While accepting that 'To err is human', the Institute of Medicine in recognizing this fatal flaw still called for a 50% reduction in the number of unexpected deaths in American hospitals [15].

The WHO estimates that 7 million surgical patients suffer significant surgical complications and 1 million die during or immediately after surgery and akin this to the maternal and neonatal survival crisis with its suggested public health intervention and educational campaign in an attempt to improve surgical safety and quality of care [5]. The surgical mortality in developing countries is 10 times higher than developed nations [9] and deaths attributed to anesthesia are 1000-fold higher, clearly demonstrating the need to improve safety in this setting [16, 17].

Its estimated that 8 million amendable deaths occurred in 2015, with 96% in low and middle income countries. The value of lost output resulted in a projected cumulative loss of $11.2 trillion in these countries during 2015–2030, with a potential economic output loss of up to 2.6% of gross domestic product (GDP) in low-income countries by 2030 [18]. Quality of care in surgery has garnered increased attention both globally, regionally and nationally [5, 19–21]. For example the introduction of guidelines for preoperative investigations for elective surgery in 2012 at the Queen Elizabeth Hospital in Barbados resulted in savings of US $40,745.50 per year, mainly due to a significant reduction in the number of full blood count and chest X-ray tests that were ordered [20]. There is therefore a strong ethical and economic case for promoting is can be reduced with the implementation of evidence-based best practice in developing countries. Following the implementation of the WHO SSC, evidence suggests it is particularly effective in a resource-poor setting. The largest decrease in complications (74.3%) was in low-income or middle-income countries [22].

3. Guidelines, checklist and protocols

Clinical practice guidelines are evidence-based recommendations for the treatment of patients with specific problems. Guidelines are developed by groups that combine people with expertise in conducting systematic reviews and health economic analyses, with those with the expertise in the clinical area (from health professionals and patients) [1]. The uptake of clinical practice guidelines has been inconsistent despite their potent to improve the quality of care and patient outcome. The WHO recommends that for each problem to be addressed by the development of guidelines, the following steps should be taken:

a. Define the specific issue to be addressed by the guidelines

b. Undertake a systematic review of the evidence available

c. Develop recommendations linked to the strength of evidence

d. Draft guidelines and for each recommendation it is best to list "highly recommended", 'recommended' or 'suggested'. These should be shared initially with all stakeholders for feedback before a final version.

e. Finally the guidelines should be tested through pilot evaluations with appropriate feedback and a full dissemination strategy implemented.

The use of guidelines usually covers common surgical problems and brings together the evidence and risks/benefits considerations for certain recommendations such that the best decisions can be made. There is still some individuality that is left to the managing team. Oftentimes guidelines are cumbersome documents of multiple pages and interpretation and implementation is made easier by a one-page summary document in simple easy to understand wording and should be readily available to all areas where patients are cared for.

Guidelines differ somewhat from protocols and checklists as here the adopted strategy should be strictly adhered to. The checklist was adapted from the field of aviation, where it was developed in response to a crash after investigations revealed the crash was as a result of a pilot failing to perform one of the steps necessary for safe takeoff [23]. Another similar area is Formula 1 racing where a high level of teamwork, focus and performance lead by team leader is necessary for optimal outcome. Meticulous training and practice is required for ideal F1 pit stop. It takes significant resources to change behavior and incorporate its use into routine daily practice [6, 7, 23]. In adjusted analysis, the use of and compliance with a checklist-based safety system was associated with a more than a 30 percent decrease in mortality and morbidity respectively [24, 25]. The decrease in surgical adverse events after implementation of checklists seems to be greater in developing countries [26] but even in well performing systems in developed countries stand to improve [27], proving that even highly skilled operating room teams need tools to help them achieve optimal results. Still it is in the low and middle income countries that the checklist use is not universally promoted or implemented, suggesting an opportunity for advocacy and education in the use of this safety tool [6].

It has been shown that the communication failures are common, affecting up to 30% of interactions in the operating room [28] and the use of a checklist may prevent more than half of the communication failures from occurring [29] by orienting the team to the individual patient, alerting each member to potential complications and encouraging team members to voice concerns when they notice an error occurring [30]. The proper use of the checklist may be a marker for teamwork and cooperation within the operating room. This calls into question whether it is the improved teamwork or the checklist. While it may be difficult to be absolutely sure of the underlying reasons for the use of checklists and improved patient outcomes, and while it is accepted that the checklist culture improves the safety culture within an institution, a firm sense of commitment is necessary, as it may become a routine activity of checking off boxes without actually driving behavior change or improvement, giving a false sense of security [31, 32]. The lack of benefit after the widespread implementation of a checklist in a hospital system is well documented and may in fact represent a more 'real world' situation [33] but also speaks to the need sometimes to modify these instruments to suite the local population.

Protocols are a set of standardized orders governing the management of a surgical problem and as such represent another means of attempting quality improvement in surgery. The development and introduction of standardized enhanced recovery and fast-track protocols in the preoperative management of surgical patients occurred over 20 years ago [34] and is well known for the benefits of reduce length of hospital stay, infection rates and costs as evidenced by various publications [35, 36]. A well-executed enhanced recovery protocol requires a multi-disciplinary team buy-in (both medical personnel and administration) and the active participation of both the patient and family. The pillars of this successful program will include the principles of carbohydrate loading, early feeding, early ambulation, goal-directed fluid therapy, and opiate-sparing analgesics. Newer anesthetic techniques, minimally invasive surgery and an emphasis on greater patient education will reduce the physiologic stress of surgical trauma and therefore less organ dysfunction. The ERAS protocols also uses evidence-based adjustments in the use of nasogastric tubes, drains, urinary catheters, preoperative bowel preparation and the use of antibiotics [37]. Although they were popularized with colorectal surgery, they have now been extended to a wide spectrum of other gastrointestinal and non-gastrointestinal surgery with maintenance of the gains [38–40].

4. Multidisciplinary meetings

The multidisciplinary approach is a concept that has been around for at least 50–60 years [41]. In fact the theoretical concept is revolutionary and as the base of medical knowledge increases the role of the single "super doctor" is now becoming obsolete. Daily hundreds of new articles filled with research done by even larger numbers of medically trained personnel enter the world of medicine. The National Health Service (NHS) defines this concept as follows: "A multidisciplinary approach involves drawing appropriately from multiple disciplines to explore problems outside of normal boundaries and reach solutions based on a new understanding of complex situations" [42]. This definition in itself is very broad but at least offers a framework in which to operate. There are some definitions used for defining the concept of the Multidisciplinary Team (MDT). According to the NHS in the UK, "a Multidisciplinary Team Meeting is defined as a care activity, a care activity referring to an individualized point of care service for patients." Furthermore, a MDT meeting is defined as, "...a meeting of the group of professionals from one or more clinical disciplines who together make decisions regarding recommended treatment of individual patients. Multidisciplinary Teams may specialize in certain conditions, such as Cancer. Clinical decisions are made based on reviews of clinical documentation such as case notes, test results, diagnostic imaging, etc. The patient may or may not be present [43].

According to specialist opinion across many surgical fields, the role of multidisciplinary teams is integral in improving patient quality care as it relates to time to time to diagnosis and treatment. There is also an economic benefit as there would be less requests for unnecessary tests therefore improving resource management [44]. In fact although there is much evidence that these multidisciplinary systems are effective in improving different parameters as it relates to different fields in medicine, the very definition of a multidisciplinary team itself is lacking. Not only is a standardized definition lacking but there is no well defined, internationally recognized set of criteria that can be used to determine if the "MDT" being assessed in each study is operating at a certain standard. It is therefore reasonable to assume that the evidence may not always point in the accurate direction due to the assessment of possibly "substandard" multidisciplinary teams littering the pool of literature. This being said, there is still overwhelming support for the use of these teams in recent literature and this is most certainly a positive indicator considering the previous point.

As mentioned before there are many advantages to the use of MDTs in clinical practice however many obstacles to their effective implementation remain. The one to one traditional clinician:patient interaction is lacking in many ways and MDTs seek to fill those gaps. One of the most obvious advantages is the sharing of knowledge across specialties. This leads to new perspectives on patient care and improved resource management as it relates to patient investigations. The multidisciplinary team meeting is a learning opportunity for specialists and this increases their exposure to evidence-based protocols and guidelines from other disciplines. One cannot fail to mention that the patient perceives this as having the benefit of a second opinion and in addition to improving the clinical intervention through consultation, may improve their perception of the quality of care they are receiving. There are also several reasons to explain the difficulty in integrating the use of multidisciplinary teams as a routine part of patient care. The ambiguity of who is needed at these meetings may lead to having not enough, or too many clinicians attending the meetings. It is an investment of time that may not be perceived as effective by some. There is an additional structure required to maintain these meetings which would mean more finances poured into human resources. If no dedicated staff for this purpose is chosen then the question of which existing department would be responsible for holding multidisciplinary meetings for which subset of patients [45].

According to the WHO in February 2015, cancer is a leading cause of morbidity and mortality worldwide, with approximately 14 million new cases and 8.2 million cancer-related deaths reported in 2012 [46]. Great interest has been generated in the application of the use of multidisciplinary teams toward the management of patients with potentially high risk and major cancer surgery [47]. In 2012, the NHS published a retrospective cohort study where breast cancer survival in intervention and non-intervention groups not treated by an MDT were compared with intervention and non-intervention groups treated by an MDT. This study found a significant decrease in mortality among the intervention group for those treated by an MDT [48]. Another example of the benefit of this application is in a retrospective cohort study done by Stephens MR et al. where a cohort of patients for R0 oesophagectomy treated by an MDT was compared with a cohort of patients treated by six individual general surgeons. A statistically significant difference in major parameters was found. Operative mortality (5.7% vs. 26%, chi2 = 8.22, P = 0.004), 5-year survival (52% vs. 10%, chi2 = 15.05, P = 0.0001) and rate of open and closed laparotomy and thoracotomy all had statistically significant improvements [49]. This is one of the very few pieces of available publications providing evidence of the utility of MDTs in high risk surgery and although encouraging, there is still more need for evidence as it relates to specific compositions of MDTs as the results may differ based on the specialists involved in the planning of these cases.

Some professionals are of the belief that a multidisciplinary team should be available for all surgical cases in order to improve the outcomes of all surgical patients who seek tertiary care. It is important to note that this may not always be an efficient use of resources. For instance, in 2015, Chien-Chou Pan et al. explored the survival rates of patients treated by an MDT for stage III and IV non-small cell lung cancer had statistically significantly higher survival rates than those not treated by an MDT. For those with stages I and II, the survival rates did not differ significantly [50]. This is an example that supports the use of multidisciplinary teams for high risk cases as the benefits may only be worth the risk in these cases.

Although the little evidence emerging thus far is in support of the implementation of MDTs, the favorable results may be partly due to flaws in study design, various biases in enrollment of participants for these studies and other factors associated with the presence of the MDT itself. For example, because this is a relatively newly explored concept, there is a lack of randomized controlled trials. Doing such studies would also raise ethical concerns especially as the MDT is already viewed by many as a higher standard of patient care and denying a patient this resource when available may be seen as questionable morally. Patients enrolled for studies for MDTs may be dependent on the referring physician and it may be reasonable to assume persons who are more likely to survive from further intervention would be in the majority of those referred to an MDT. It is also important not to forget that when a patient is referred to an MDT, they may have several investigations

Targets/goals	Suggested intervention
Establish baseline practice at the local institution	Audit of current practice
Identify barriers to implementation	Interviews & surveys: surgeons, nurse anesthetists, residents, physicians
Identify relevant interventions	Systematic review of the literature
Develop guidelines and protocols based on evidence and consensus	Modified Delphi method, both evidence & expert opinion incorporated

Table 1.
Implementation of guidelines/checklist/protocols.

expedited that would have otherwise not have been done or would have taken longer to be completed. These factors are all important to consider in interpretation of increased survival rates seen in the existing literature.

Overall, it is evident that the presence of the multidisciplinary team has been beneficial for specific patient populations. Whether this benefit is directly as a result of the team itself or the associated factors such as decreased time to investigations or other similar factors may not necessarily be of significant concern. As this topic continues to be explored in the literature and is also being applied in increasing numbers of patient care institutions, we will continue to learn about the utility of these teams both in a general sense and as it relates to more specific patient populations (**Table 1**).

4.1 What are the barriers to implementation?

Providing optimal care to patients based on the best evidence is difficult as the half-life of knowledge is estimated to be approximately 3–5 years therefore it is very difficult for physicians to keep up with the medical literature. Multiple strategies are often required to make changes and provide optimal care. Knowledge translation is a dynamic and iterative process that includes synthesis and dissemination of the best available evidence in an ethically sound manner to improve health, provide more effective health services and products and strengthen the healthcare system. It requires collaboration between multiple stakeholders and multifaceted interventions such as audits and feedback, reminders, educational strategies, decision aids and standardized orders. Physicians usually play a leading role in implementation as they are usually opinion leaders. Additionally they are well respected and trusted by all members of the health care team. Especially in developing countries where there is a lot to be gained some answers may lie outside the physician or hospital. Measures such as legislation, public education and advocacy, revision of the medical curriculum, patient handbooks and other health promotional material may all have a role in eliciting change in behavior. Varying committed members of the health care team may have to assume the role of the opinion leader or 'champion'. Recommendations are more likely to be followed if they are simple, inclusive, with a high level of evidence but are more likely to succeed with an evaluative component and with rewards and disincentives.

5. Conclusions

The modern surgical environment is complex with multiple components perhaps too much to be considered for any one individual. The dynamic nature of medical knowledge in an environment of an informed patient dictates that consumers of health care in a globalized world expect the best outcome. A multidisciplinary approach using the best available evidence is just the first step in knowledge translation. The entire health system may need to change. This is the active process of implementation among the multiple stakeholders that will be necessary to effect change. The combination of a multidisciplinary team using guidelines or protocols aided by checklists is one way of ensuring quality in the surgical health care system. Consideration can also be given to a rewards and disincentives packages as we seek to change behavior. Of course, once implemented and with appropriate audits, we should see positive results, that is, improved quality care. We recognize that this is a dynamic process, with active monitoring of the literature for emerging/changing evidence, and revisions at designated intervals as necessary.

Author details

Joseph Martin Plummer*, Mark S. Newnham and Timothy Henry
Department of Surgery, Radiology, Anesthesia and Intensive Care,
University of the West Indies, Kingston, Jamaica

*Address all correspondence to: joseph.plummer02@uwimona.edu.jm

IntechOpen

References

[1] Alderson P, Tan T. The use of Cochrane reviews in NICE clinical guidelines. Cochrane Database of Systematic Reviews. 9 Aug 2011;**12**:ED000032. DOI: 10.1002/14651858.ED000032

[2] Schmid O, Chalmers L, Berexnicki L. Evidence-to-practice gaps in the management of community-dwelling Australian patients with ischaemic heart disease. Journal of Clinical Pharmacy and Therapeutics. 2015;**40**(4):398-403

[3] Ingraham AH, Cohen ME, Billimoria KY, Dimick JB, Richards KE, et al. Association of surgical care improvement project infection-related process measure compliance with risk-adjusted outcomes: Implications for quality measurement. Journal of the American College of Surgeons. 2010;**211**(6):705-714

[4] Cohen ME, Liu Y, Ko CY, Hall BL. Improved surgical outcomes for ACS NSQIP hospitals over time: Evaluation of hospitals cohorts with up to 8 years of participation. Annals of Surgery. 2016;**263**(2):267-273

[5] World Alliance for Patient Safety. WHO Guidelines for Safe Surgery 2009: Safe Surgery Saves Lives. Geneva: World Health Organization; 2009

[6] Weiser TG, Haynes AB. Ten years of the surgical safety checklist. British Journal of Surgery. Jul 2018;**105**(8):927-929

[7] Gawande AA. From cowboys to pit crews: Patient focused care starts with a team approach. In: ACS Clinical Congress News; Wed Oct 24. 2018. p. 1. Available from: ACSCNEWS.ORG

[8] Hall BL, Hamilton BH, Richards K, Billimoria KY, Cohen ME, Ko CY. Does surgical quality in the American College of Surgeons National Surgery Quality Improvement Program: An evaluation of all hospitals. Annals of Surgery. 2009;**250**(3):363-376

[9] Weiser TG, Regenbogen SE, Thompson KD, et al. An estimation of the global volume of surgery: A modelling strategy based on available data. Lancet. 2008;**372**:139-144

[10] Bainbridge D, Martin J, Arango M, Cheng D. Evidence-based perioperative clinical outcomes research (EPiCOR) group. Lancet. 2012;**380**(9847):1075-1081

[11] Sokol DK, Wilson J. What is a surgical complication. World Journal of Surgery. 2008;**32**(6):942-944

[12] Gross M. Reporting complications on a general surgical service. Canadian Journal of Surgery. 2000;**43**(2):86

[13] Brennan TA, Leape LL, Laird NM, Hebert L, Localio AR, Lawthers AG, et al. Incidence of adverse events and negligence in hospitalized patients. Results of the Harvard Medical Practice Study I. The New England Journal of Medicine. 1991;**324**(6):370-376

[14] Treadwell JR, Lucas S, Tsou AY. Surgical checklists: A systematic review of impacts and implementation. BMJ Quality and Safety. 2014;**23**(4):299-318

[15] Russell T. Safety and quality improvement in surgical practice. Annals of Surgery. 2006;**244**(5):653-655

[16] Ouro-Bang'na Maman AF, Tomta K, Ahouangbévi S, Chobli M. Deaths associated with anaesthesia in Togo, West Africa. Tropical Doctor. 2005;**35**:220-222

[17] Li G, Warner M, Lang BH, Huang L, Sun LS. Epidemiology

of anesthesia-related mortality in the United States, 1999-2005. Anesthesiology. 2009;**110**:759-765

[18] Alkire BC, Peters AW, Shrime MG, Meara JG. The economic consequences of mortality amendable to high-quality health care in low and middle-income countries. Health Affairs (Millwood). 2018;**37**(6):988-996

[19] Rogers SO. The holy grail of surgical quality improement: Process measures of risk-adjusted outcomes? The American Surgeon. 2006;**72**(11):1046-1050

[20] Nicholls J, Gaskin PS, Ward J, Areti YK. Guidelines for preoperative investigations for elective surgery at Queen Elizabeth Hospital: Effects on practices, outcomes, and costs. Journal of Clinical Anesthesia. 2016;**35**:176-189

[21] Plummer JM, Williams N, Leake PA, Ferron-Boothe D, Meeks-Aitken N, Mitchell DI, et al. Surgical quality in colorectal cancer. Annals of Medicine and Surgery (London). 2015;**5**:52-56

[22] Vivekanantham S, Ravindran RP, Shanmugarajah K, Maruthappu M, Shalhoub J. Surgical safety checklists in developing countries. International Journal of Surgery. 2014;**12**(1):2-6

[23] Gawande A. The Checklist Manifesto: How to Get Things Right. 1st ed. New York, NY: Metropolitan Books; 2010

[24] de Vries EN, Prins HA, Crolla RM, den Outer AJ, van Andel G, van Helden SH, et al. Effect of a comprehensive surgical safety system on patients outcome. The New England Journal of Medicine. 2010;**363**:1928-1937

[25] Birkmeyer JD. Strategies for improving surgical quality-checklists and beyond. The New England Journal of Medicine. 2010;**363**:1963-1965

[26] de Jager E, McKenna C, Bartlett L, Gunnarsson R, Ho YH. Post-operative adverse events inconsistently improved by the World Health Organization surgical safety checklist: A systematic literature review of 25 studies. World Journal of Surgery. 2016;**40**(8):1842-1858

[27] Haynes AB, Edmondson L, Lipsitz SR, Molina G, Neville BA, Singer SJ, et al. Mortality trends after a voluntary checklist-based surgical safety collaborative. Annals of Surgery. 2017;**266**:923-929

[28] Hu YY, Arriaga AF, Peyre SE, Corso KA, Roth EM, Greenberg CC. Deconstructing intraoperative communication failures. The Journal of Surgical Research. 2012;**177**(1):37-42

[29] Hendrickson SE, Wadhera RK, Elbardissi AW, Wiegmann DA, Sundt TM. 3rd development and pilot evaluation of a preoperative briefing protocol for cardiovascular surgery. Journal of the American College of Surgeons. 2009;**208**(6):1115-1123

[30] Pugel AE, Simianu VV, Flum DR, Dellinger EP. Use of surgical checklist ti improve communication and reduce complications. Journal of Infection and Public Health. 2015;**8**(3):219-225

[31] Levy SM, Senter CE, Hawkins RB, Zhao JY, Doody K, Kao LS, et al. Implementing a surgical checklist: More than ckecking a box. Surgery. 2012;**152**(3):331-336

[32] Putman LR, Levy SM, Sajid M, Bubuisson DA, Rogers NB, Kao LS, et al. Multifaceted interventions improve adherence to the surgical checklist. Surgery. 2014;**156**(2):336-344

[33] Ubach DR, Govindarajan A, Saskin R, Wilton AS, Baxter NN. Introduction of surgical safety checklist in Ontario, Canada. The New England Journal of Medicine. 2014;**370**(11):1029-1038

[34] Kim BJ, Aloia TA. What is "enhanced recovery" and how can I do it? Journal of Gastrointestinal Surgery. 2018;**22**(1):164-171

[35] Lassen K, Soop M, Nygren J, Cox PB, Hendry PO, Spies C, et al. Consensus review of optimal preoperative care in colorectal surgery. Enhanced Recovery After Surgery (ERAS) Group recommendations. Archives of Surgery. 2009;**144**: 961-969

[36] Zhuang CL, Ye XZ, Zhang XD, Chen BC, Yu Z. Enhanced recovery after surgery programs versus traditional care for colorectal surgery: Meta-analysis of randomized trials. Diseases of the Colon and Rectum. 2013;**56**(5):667-678

[37] Kehlet H. Fast-track colorectal surgery. Lancet. 2008;**371**:791-793

[38] Parizh D, Ascher E, Raza Rizvi SA, Hingorani A, Amaturo M, Johnson E. Quality improvement initiative: Preventative surgical site infection protocol in vascular surgery. Vascular. 2018;**26**(1):47-53

[39] Bond-Smith G, Belgaumkar AP, Davidson BR, Gurusamy KS. Enhanced recovery protocols for major upper gastrointestinal, liver and pancreatic surgery. Cochrane Database of Systematic Reviews. 2016;**2**:CD011382

[40] Ryan SL, Sen A, Staggers K, Luerssen TG, Jea A. Texas Children's Hospital Spine Study Group. Journal of Neurosurgery. Pediatrics. 2014;**14**(3):259-265

[41] Patkar V, Acosta D, Davidson T, Jones A, Fox J, Keshtgar M. Cancer multidisciplinary team meetings: Evidence, challenges, and the role of clinical decision support technology. International Journal of Breast Cancer. 2011;**2011**:7. Article ID: 831605. DOI: 10.4061/2011/831605

[42] England.nhs.uk. 2018. Available from: https://www.england.nhs.uk/wp-content/uploads/2015/01/mdt-dev-guid-flat-fin.pdf [Accessed: November 28, 2018]

[43] Supporting Information: Multidisciplinary Team Meeting [Internet]. Datadictionary.nhs.uk. 2018. Available from: https://www.datadictionary.nhs.uk/data_dictionary/nhs_business_definitions/m/multidisciplinary_team_meeting_de.asp?shownav=1 [Accessed: November 28, 2018]

[44] Güler SA, Cantürk NZ. Multidisciplinary breast cancer teams and proposed standards. Ulusal cerrahi dergisi. **2014**;(1):39-41. DOI: 10.5152/UCD.2014.2724

[45] Carter S, Garside P, Black A. Multidisciplinary team working, clinical networks, and chambers; opportunities to work differently in the NHS. BMJ Quality & Safety. 2003;**12**:i25-i28

[46] World Health Organization (WHO). Cancer Factsheet Number 297. 2015. Available from: http://www.who.int/mediacentre/factsheets/fs297/en/

[47] Ziabari Y, Wigmore T, Kasivisvanathan R. The multidisciplinary team approach for high-risk and major cancer surgery. BJA Education. 2017;**17**(8):255-261. DOI: 10.1093/bjaed/mkx003

[48] Kesson Eileen M, Allardice Gwen M, David GW, Burns Harry JG, Morrison David S. Effects of multidisciplinary team working on breast cancer survival: Retrospective, comparative, interventional cohort study of 13 722 women. BMJ. 2012;**344**:e27149

[49] Stephens MR, Lewis WG, Brewster AE, et al. Multidisciplinary team management is associated with improved outcomes after surgery for

esophageal cancer. Diseases of the Esophagus. 2006;**19**:164-171

[50] Pan CC, Kung PT, Wang YH, Chang YC, Wang ST, Tsai WC. Effects of multidisciplinary team care on the survival of patients with different stages of non-small cell lung cancer: A national cohort study. PLoS One. 2015;**10**(5):e0126547. DOI: 10.1371/journal.pone.0126547

Chapter 5

Inhospital Outcome of Elderly Patients in an Intensive Care Unit in a Sub-Saharan Hospital

Martin Lankoande, Papougnezambo Bonkoungou,

Oubian Soulemane, Ghislain Somda and Joachim Sanou

Abstract

People living more and more longer and elderly is growing and that requires change in health system including geriatric care to be innovative. The aim of this study was to analyze causes and prognosis of older patients admitted in an intensive care unit (ICU) in Sub-Sahara area. A retrospective study over 5 years of patients aged 65 years and above admitted in ICU of Yalgado Ouedraogo was carried out. Of the 2116 patients admitted in ICU, 237 (11.2%) were older. The mean age was 71.7 ± 6.1 years. Males were predominant (sex ratio = 2.4). Medical history was present in 80.6%. The Charlson mean score was 4.8 ± 1.8. Patients with coma represented 42%. Ambulatory Simplified Acute Physiologic Score (ASAPS) up to 8 was recorded in 49%. Medical diseases (60%) like nervous system (37.9%) were reported. Stroke and general surgery were the main affection. Globally treatment was based on fluid management and oxygen supply. During ICU stay, complications occurred in 37.5% like acute respiratory distress syndrome (ARDS) in 10.5%. The mean length of stay was 5.3 ± 7.4 days. The elderly mortality was 73%; those 90% died within 7 days. In multivariate analysis, shock (odds ratio: OR = 2.2, p = 0.002), severe brain trauma (OR = 9.6, p = 0.002), coma (OR 5.8 p < 0.003), surgical condition (OR = 4.2, p = 0.003), ASAPS ≥ 8 (OR = 4.3, p = 0.001), complication occurring (OR = 5.2, p = 0.001), and stroke (OR = 3.7, p = 0.001) were independent risk factors of death. Elderly patients are frequently admitted in ICU with high mortality.

Keywords: elderly, intensive care unit, mortality, Burkina Faso

1. Introduction

People aged 65 or 60 years and above are considered older [1], respectively, in developed countries and in Africa [1]. The world population grows older in most regions. In the year 2012, the global population reached 7 billion, and 562 (8%) millions of them were older. In 2015, the elderly rose by 55 million representing 8.5% of the world population [2]. In Africa, the rate of elderly (6.6% in 2015) will reach 9.6% in 2050 [2]. Like in other countries older people are increasing in Burkina Faso. This demographic transition increase health care needs especially healthcare facilities, policies and training. Critical patients have increased risk because of associated morbidities [3]. These people are characterized by their frailty with risk of death. This high risk met in anesthesia and intensive care raises some voice around the world particularly in the UK where some actions like implementation of perioperative medicine were planned. The physician has a major role for health-care improvement for multimorbid and frail patients [4]. In Burkina Faso, intensive care services need to be implemented. Government-adopted politics and some physicians are in specialization in foreign countries. No guidelines are available on older patient care in our countries, and patients are treated like other patients. More and more older patients are admitted in ICU and most died. In order to reduce the number of deaths, more information need to be identified for a better evidence-based action. The aim of this study was to analyze causes and prognosis of older patients admitted in the ICU of Yalgado Hospital in Burkina Faso.

2. Methods and materials

2.1 Setting and population

A retrospective study was carried out among patients aged ≥65 years in the ICU of the teaching hospital Yalgado Ouedraogo over 5 years (January 1, 2011– December 31, 2015). The Yalgado Ouédraogo Hospital is 800-bedded hospital where no specialist in geriatric is available. The ICU is an 8-bedded unit and is poorly equipped. Data recorded after approval by the Ethical and Research Committee (Ethical and National Scientific Research and Technology Center, ENSRTC) include sociodemographic, comorbidities, diagnosis, causes of ICU admission, Glasgow Coma Score, the Ambulatory Simplified Acute Physiologic Score (ASAPS), Charlson Comorbidity Score, sepsis, shock on admission, length of stay (LOS), management, and outcome. The ASAPS [5] is a scale used for gravity evaluation for ICU patients. Patients were categorized into three groups of age (65–74 years or "young old," 75–84 or "old old," and >85 or oldest old).

2.2 Statistical analysis

Quantitative data were presented as mean and standard deviation. Their variations were analyzed using ANOVA test. Qualitative data are presented as numbers and percentages and variations analyzed using the chi-square test. Chi-square test helped to compare survivors to non-survivors with $p \leq 0.05$. Analysis was performed with the Epidemiologic Info package 7.1.5.0.

3. Results

Among 2116 patients admitted in ICU, 237 (11.2%) were older. The mean age was 71.7 ± 6.1 years; the sex ratio was 2.4. A total of 173 deaths were observed (73%). Demographic and facility characteristics of deaths of patients are summarized in **Table 1**.

Comorbidity was identified in 80.6%. The Charlson mean score was 4.79 ± 1.83 [IC 95%; 2–12]. The mean score of Glasgow scale was 4.8 ± 1.2. Medical history and comorbidity are described in **Table 2**. Among the patients, 42% were admitted with coma. The ASAPS ≥8 was recorded as 49%. Clinical data are summarized in **Table 3**. Medical condition (60%) and nervous disease (37.9%) were the main diagnosis. Neurology disease and general surgery were the main affection by specialty (**Figure 1**). Stroke was the most frequent (27.4%) followed by peritonitis (**Table 3**). Intensive care was based on fluid, pain killers, and oxygen supply.

Characteristic		Frequency	Percentage
Age (years)	65–74 years	167	70.5
	75–84 years	58	24.5
	More 84 years	12	5
Gender	Male	167	70.5
	Female	70	29.5
Residency	Urban	159	67.1
	Rural area	78	32.9
Profession	Retired	48	32.6
	Housewife	37	25.2
	Farmer	31	21.1
	Public/private	31	21.1
Referral facilities	District hospital	107	45.1
	Regional hospital	39	16.5
	Dispensary	3	1.3
	Teaching hospital[a]	19	8
	Private hospital	69	29.1

[a]*Teaching Hospital (YO: 8; Blaise Compaoré Hospital: 6; Sourou Sanou Hospital = 5).*

Table 1.
Demographic characteristics of patients (n = 237).

Medical history		Frequency	Percentage
High blood pressure		120	50.6
Diabetes		56	23.6
Ulcer		15	6.3
Heart disease		9	3.8
Kidney failure		8	3.4
Stroke		4	1.7
Asthma		4	1.7
HIV/AIDS		3	1.3
Lymphoma		2	0.8
Live cancer		2	0.8
Esophagus stenosis		1	0.4
Esophagitis		1	0.4
Liver abscess		1	0.4
Goiter disease		1	0.4
None		60	25.3
Charlson score	<3	25	10.5
	4–5	139	58.6
	6–7	53	22.3
	≥8	20	8.4

Table 2.
Past history and comorbidity (N = 237).

Clinical data	Number	Percentage
Admission condition		
Medical condition	183	77.2
Surgical condition	54	22.8
Diseases		
Stroke	65	27.4
Prostate tumor	27	11.4
Sepsis	26	10.9
Trauma/burn	25	10.5
Bowel obstruction	13	5.5
Heart disease	18	2.5
Diabetic acute metabolic complications	20	8.4
Kidney failure	16	6.7
Other[a]	27	11.4
Total	237	100
Complications		
Sepsis	25	10.5
Acute respiratory distress syndrome	38	42.7
Shock	15	6.3
Coma	19	21.3
Bed sores	8	3.4
Acute pulmonary edema	5	2.1
Pulmonary aspiration	5	2.1
Pulmonary embolism	1	0.4
Other[b]	5	2.1
Outcomes		
Death in ICU	173	73
Transfer to other ward	48	20.2
Hospital discharge with physician authorization	10	4.2
Discharge without physician authorization	6	2.5
Total	237	100

[a]*Other: anemia (n = 3), dehydratation (n = 2);* [b]*Hernia, blood disorder, ulcer, hydronephrosis, asthma, skin disease, leukemia.*

Table 3.
Diagnosis and outcome of patients (n = 237).

During hospitalization, complications occurred in 37.5%, and ARDS was the most frequent (10.5%). In total, 173 older patients died (73%). The length of stay was 5.3 ± 7.4 days [IC 95%; 1 58] (**Table 4**).

Most patients were between 64 and 74 years old. There was significant difference in terms of group of age, between patients with a Charlson score up to 8 versus less than 8 (p = 0.001) and those with complications occurring in ICU versus no

Psychiatric ▪ 2
SKIN/IST ▪ 2
Gynecolgy-Obstetric ▪ 2
ENT ▬ 4
Infectiology ▬ 5
Digestive ▬▬ 8
Traumatology ▬▬▬▬▬▬▬▬ 24
Cardiology ▬▬▬▬▬ 15
Pneumology ▬▬▬▬▬▬ 18
Nephrology ▬▬▬▬▬▬ 19
Neurosurgery ▬▬▬▬▬▬ 20
Urology ▬▬▬▬▬▬▬ 21
Endocrinology ▬▬▬▬▬▬▬ 23
General surgery ▬▬▬▬▬▬▬▬▬▬▬▬▬▬▬▬ 55
Neurology ▬▬▬▬▬▬▬▬▬▬▬▬▬▬▬▬▬▬▬ 70

0   10   20   30   40   50   60   70   80

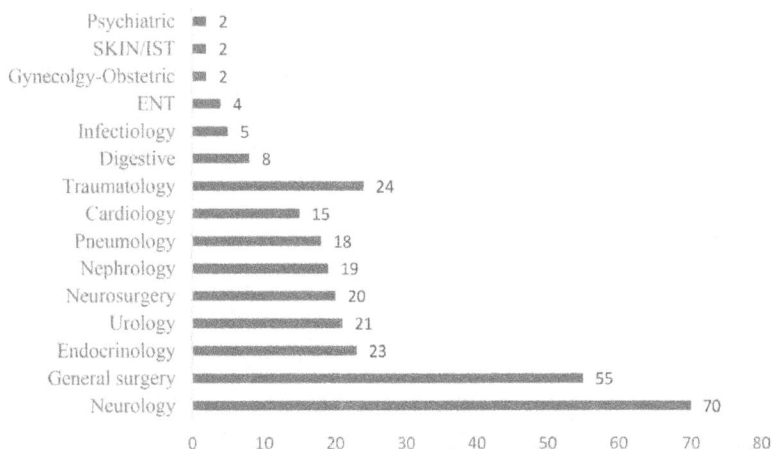

Figure 1.
Nature of disease (n = 237).

Characteristics	All patients (N = 237)	Non-survivors (n = 173)	Survivors (n = 64)	P value
Age (mean; years)	71.7 ± 6.1	71.6 ± 5.9	72.1 ± 6.4	0.5
Age group (%)				
65–74	167 (70.4)	123 (73.6)	44 (26.3)	0.7
75–84	58 (24.5)	42 (72.4)	16 (27.6)	0.9
85 above	12 (5.1)	8 (66.6)	4 (33.3)	0.6
Gender				
Male (n = 167)	167 (70.4)	127 (76.05)	40 (23.9)	0.1
Female (n = 70)	70 (29.6)	46 (65.7)	24 (34.3)	
Residency area				
Urban	159 (67.1)	97 (61)	62 (39)	0.3
Rural	78 (32.9)	62 (79.5)	16 (20.5)	
Reference specialty (%)				
Emergency service	134 (56.4)	108 (80.6)	26 (20.4)	0.001
Medicine	21 (8.8)	14 (66.6)	7 (33.8)	0.4
Surgery	54 (22.8)	49 (90.7)	5 (9.3)	0.003
Reasons for admission				
ACS	133 (56.1)	109 (81.9)	24 (18)	<0.001
Poor condition	6 (2.5)	3 (50)	3 (50)	0.3
Burn	11 (4.6)	7 (63.64)	4 (36.4)	0.4
ARDS	9 (3.8)	7 (77.7)	2 (22.2)	1
Shock	78 (32.9)	47 (60.3)	31 (39.7)	0.002
Charlson score (Median)	4.8 ± 1.8	4.6 ± 1.7	5.09 ± 2.04	0.12
≥ 8	20 (8.4)	11 (55)	9 (45)	0.03
< 8	217 (91.6)	103 (47.4)	76 (52.6)	0.4
Glasgow coma score (mean value)	9.64 ± 4.01	8.9 ± 3.8	11.8 ± 3.6	0.03
< 8	42.06	69 (88.4)	9 (11.5)	<0.001
≥ 8	57.9	58 (68.2)	76 (31.8)	
ASAPS (mean)	7.9 ± 3.5	8.6 ± 3.5	5.8 ± 2.6	<0.001
ASAPS ≥8		150 (87)	13	
ASAPS <8		109 (63.5)	36.6	
Diagnosis				
Stroke	65 (27.4)	57 (87.69)	8 (12.31)	0.001

Characteristics	All patients (N = 237)	Non-survivors (n = 173)	Survivors (n = 64)	P value
Peritonitis	22 (9.3)	18 (81.82)	4 (18.18)	0.4
AMCD[A]	20 (8.4)	10 (50)	10 (50)	0.01
SBT[B]	19 (8)	18 (94.74)	1 (5.26)	0.02
Bowel obstruction	13 (5.5)	7 (53.85)	6 (46.15)	0.1
Burn	10 (4.2)	6 (60)	4 (40)	0.4
Severe infection	10 (4.2)	8 (80)	2 (2)	0.7
Prostatic adenoma	9 (3.8)	5 (55.56)	4 (44.44)	0.2
Heart disease	6 (2.5)	4 (66.67)	2 (33.33)	0.6
Prostatic cancer	5 (2.1)	1 (20)	4 (80)	0.01
Inguinal hernia	5 (2.1)	3 (60)	2 (40)	0.6
Other[C]	53 (22.4)	36 (67.92)	17 (32.0)	0.1
Complications occurred in ICU				
Yes = 89	89 (37.5)	80 (89.9)	9 (10.1)	<0.001
No = 148	148 (62.5)	93 (62.8)	55 (37.2)	
Mechanical ventilation	2 (0.8)	2 (100)	0	Ki = 0.7
Length of stay (mean)	5.3 ± 7.4	5.2 ± 8	5.5 ± 5.1	0.8

ACS, alteration of consciousness; ARDS, acute respiratory distress syndrome, [A]AMCD, acute metabolic complication of diabetes; [B]SBT, severe brain trauma, [C]Other disease, ASAPS: ambulatory simplified acute physiologic scale.

Table 4.
Comparison of survivors and non-survivor's patients (n = 237).

Variables	65–74 years n = 167 (70.4%)	75–84 years n = 58 (24.5%)	Over 84 years n = 12 (5.1%)	P value
Age (mean; years)	68.3 ± 2.8	78.2 ± 2.5	86.6 ± 1.6	<0.001
Gender				
Male (n = 167)	118	40	9	0.9
Female (n = 70)	49	18	3	
Reasons for admission				
ACS	92	33	6	0.9
Poor condition	68	26	5	0.6
Burn	7	2	1	0.7
ARDS	13	6	0	0.4
Shock	11	4	2	0.4
Charlson score	4.5	5.1	6.3	0.001
≥ 8	12	5	3	0.1
< 8	155	53	9	
Glasgow score (mean)	9.7 ± 4.02	9.4 ± 4.1	8.8 ± 3.5	0.6
< 8	12	5	3	0.1
≥ 8	155	53	9	
ASAPS (Mean)	7.9 ± 3.8	8.08 ± 2.9	8.1 ± 2.7	0.9
ASAPS ≥8	65	25	8	0.1
ASAPS <8	77	22	4	0.4
Complications in ICU				0.01
Yes = 89	65	19	5	0.6
No = 148	102	39	7	
Mechanical ventilation	2	0	0	0.6
Length of stay (LOS)	5.3 ± 6.8	5.6 ± 9.2	2.7 ± 2.2	0.4
Death	123 (73.6)	42 (72.4)	8 (66.6)	0.2

ACS, Alteration of consciousness; ARDS, Acute respiratory distress syndrome; ICU, Intensive care unit; ASAPS, Ambulatory simplified acute physiologic scale.

Table 5.
Comparison of patients according to age group (n = 237).

Diagnosis	Adjusted OR (CI 95%)	p
Medical condition without coma	Reference	
Surgery	4.2 [2.4–10.3]	0.003
Coma at admission	2.9 [1.6–5.4]	0.001
Coma in ICU	5.8 [2.3–14.6]	0.001
Shock during admission	2.2 [1.6–4.0]	0.002
ASAPS ≥8	4.3 [1.1–8.5]	0.001
Stroke	3.7 [1.6–8.7]	0.001
Severe brain trauma	9.6 [1.2–75.1]	0.02
Complications in ICU		0.001
No	Reference	
Yes	5.2 [2.4–11.3]	0.001

ACS, alteration of consciousness; ARDS, acute respiratory distress syndrome; ICU, intensive care unit; ASAPS, ambulatory simplified acute physiologic scale.

Table 6.
Risk factors for ICU mortality of elderly patients.

complications occurring (p = 0.01) (**Table 5**). In multivariate analysis, surgery, coma, shock, stroke, and severe brain trauma were independent risks factors of death (**Table 6**).

4. Discussion

Older patients accounted for 11.2% of ICU admission. This rate is comparable to the 10% of Owojuyigbe et al. [6] findings in Nigeria but less than the findings in the United States (42–52%). Better health-care system organization, life expectancy improvement explains high prevalence in developed countries. In Burkina Faso, the elderly accounted 2.4% of the population [7]. Elderly mortality (73%) is high compared to Belayachi et al. [8] reports (44.7%) in Morocco and Wade et al. [9] (42.8%) at Senegal. The high mortality reported in developing countries compared to developed countries may be due to inadequate care, late consultation, poverty, and poor equipment of ICU.

The mean age (71.7) in this study was comparable to Owojuyigbe et al. [6] report (73 years) and Belayachi et al. [8] report (72 years). In Porto, Abelha et al. [10] reported 64.1 years. The age varies according to regions and studies. Patients were mostly males, but there is no correlation between gender and outcome in this study. In other studies, [8], [10] report similar finding, while Fowler et al. reported higher mortality with female patient [11]. In this study, the majority lives in urban area (67.1%) and was retired (32.6%). Patients were referred from district hospital (45.1%). In Burkina Faso, district hospitals are so far to the National Referral Hospital, and patients travel so far in poor condition that causes delay to care and worsens prognosis. In our study, 49.4% had high Charlson comorbidity score. Older patients have many comorbidities which reduce their capability, increase disability, decrease quality of life, and increase risk of death [12]. In the literature, it has been reported that the pooled mortality risk for elderly people with multimorbidity was high compared with those with one chronic disease or none [12, 13]. Alteration of consciousness was found in 56.1% and shock in 32.9%. Our findings were comparable to those reported by Vosylius et al. [14]. ASAPS ≥8 was recorded in 49%. The delay to consult and care worsens patient condition. Medical condition was the main diagnosis, and stroke was most frequent (27.4%) followed by peritonitis. Our findings are different with Belayachi et al. [8] who found that respiratory infections were most predominant. Diagnoses vary according to study, social environment, and countries [6, 8, 11, 14].

Advanced age alone does not preclude successful outcome [9]. In multivariate analysis, independent risk factors were surgical conditions, coma, shock during admission, ASAPS ≥8, stroke, and severe brain trauma. These findings are comparable to literature reports [9, 3, 15]. There is no difference between age groups in terms of mortality. The mean LOS was short, while 46.6% of patients died within 3 days and 90% of patient died within a week. For patients over 84 years, LOS was shorter, and inhospital mortality was less than in patients aged less than 84 years. The family usually refuse care and discharge once a poor outcome is pronounced. This explains the relatively low mortality rate and short stay of this group of

age. Elderly patients living in rural area die more than those in urban area, but this rate is not significant. The overall poor outcomes may be due to late consultation and poor quality of care due to the inadequate facilities and equipment and lack of medications due to poverty. Even most of our patients live in urban area and was retired care are not generally provided continuously because of financial barrier. Retired people do not have insurance in public hospital but only in private sector which does not have ICU. Delay to consultation may be related to limited education, traditional healing practice, poverty, and poor transportation. In Africa elderly consider conventional medicine as for infant and their family geriatric disease is associated to end of live. That sometime delay use of conventional medicine. The LOS was short in our study compared to other study (Belayachi et al. [8], 6.6 days; Fuchs et al., 9 days), but some authors found a longer LOS (12.9–23 days) [10, 16]. In our study mortality was high (73%) compared to literature [10, 11, 14, 15]. Comorbidity, frailty, low number of physicians and nurses, insufficiency of skills, lack of equipment, and insurance are some hypotheses to explain mortality. Geriatric training implementation, a good follow-up, and perioperative medicine implementation can reduce admission in ICU. In order to improve elderly care, we need to make policies, sensitize people for early consultation, and implement universal health coverage. Our study showed that most patients have comorbidities. Multimorbidity is especially common among older adults, and its negative consequences include higher disability, decrease in quality of life, and increased risk of death. The insufficiency of follow-up, limitation of skills on geriatric care, and insufficiency of hospital equipment increase risk of death.

Most of the people of Burkina Faso live in the rural area and are farmers. Cultural and financial barriers are most important in this area where people practice traditional healing because they consult later to modern health services. Diagnosis is mostly performed at an advanced condition where treatment is compromised. So the universal health coverage is not implemented, and people have to make direct payment before care. Even with most people who are living in the urban area and retried, the social security of our country does not give possibility of prepayment but only reimbursement and this situation delay care. In response to the recommendations of the World Health Organization and United Nations Assembly on Aging, our country made policies and defines laws to protect older people in the year 2015, but these laws are still unimplemented because of the lack of decree. By promoting specialization in geriatry, implementation of policies protecting older people, Burkina Faso government demonstrated a will to promote elderly well-being and health care. The national program of social protection of older people initiated in 2016 will improve health care with a better follow, universal health promotion. In the particular case of intensive care services, the national society of anesthesiology must implement perioperative medicine course. More commitment and investment are needed to enhance of the elderly care. This study has limitations due to retrospective character and long-term outcome data missing. The impact of hospitalization, biologic abnormality, the APACHE, and SOFA score on outcome was not evaluated. This study showed that most of those who live in urban area raise an issue of representativeness for the population, and we cannot generalize these findings.

5. Conclusions

Older patients were frequently admitted in the ICU of Yalgado hospital. Patients are mostly "young old" but have comorbidities. Patients were admitted with the serious condition. LOS was short which indirectly means poor management with early death. Mortality is high. The main factors of death are shock, severe brain trauma, coma, surgical condition, complication occurring, and stroke. The public must be sensitized to consult early and respect medical advices. Health-care worker must improve their skills and adapted care to older people. The implementation of geriatric center can allow improved care for a low rate of death.

Conflict of interest

None.

Notes/thanks/other declarations

Thanks to Dr. Ghislain for data collection.

Author details

Martin Lankoande[1*], Papougnezambo Bonkoungou[2], Oubian Soulemane[1], Ghislain Somda[3] and Joachim Sanou[2]

1 Regional Hospital of Koudougou, Burkina Faso

2 Teaching Hospital Yalgado Ouedraogo, Burkina Faso

3 Distric Hôpital of Gayérie, Burkina Faso

*Address all correspondence to: m.hamtaani@gmail.com

IntechOpen

References

[1] Naja S, Mohei M, Din E, Abdul M, Chehab H. An ageing world of the 21st century: A literature review. International Journal Of Community Medicine And Public Health. 2017;**4**(12):4363-4369

[2] Bureau USC. An Aging World: 2015 International Population Reports. March 2016

[3] Fuchs L, Novack V, Mclennan S, Celi LA, Baumfeld Y, Park S, et al. Trends in severity of illness on ICU admission and mortality among the elderly. PLoS One. 2014;**9**(4):1-11

[4] Burkina Faso AN. Loi n°024-2016/an. Loi. 2016

[5] Dia NM, Diallo I, Manga NM, Diop SA, Fortes-Deguenonvo L, Lakhe NA, et al. Intérêt de l'indice de gravité simplifié ambulatoire (IGSA) appliqué à des patients admis dans l'unité de soins intensifs (USI) d'un service de pathologie infectieuse à Dakar. Bulletin de la Societe de Pathologie Exotique. 2015;**108**(3):175-180

[6] Owojuyigbe AM, Adenekan AT, Babalola RN, Adetoye AO, Olateju SOA, Akonoghrere UO. Pattern and Outcome of Elderly Admissions into the Intensive Care Unit (ICU) of a Low Resource Tertiary Hospital. East and Central African Journal of Surgery. 2016;**21**(2):40-46. ISSN: 2073-9990

[7] INSD; Burkina Faso. La population du Burkina Faso. 2009

[8] Belayachi J, El M, Dendane T, Abidi K, Abouqal R, Zeggwagh AA. Factors predicting mortality in elderly patients admitted to a Moroccan medical intensive care unit. Southern African Journal of Critical Care. 2018;**28**(1):1-12

[9] Barsaoui S, Siaka K, Ouattara A, Soro D, Okon JB, Assi C, et al. Devenir des sujets âgés en réanimation à Dakar (Sénégal) Outcome of elderly patients

in an intensive care unit in Dakar, Senegal. Medecine et Sante Tropicales. 2012;**22**(2):223-224

[10] Abelha F, Maia P, Landeiro N, Neves A, Barros H. Determinants of outcome in patients admitted to a surgical intensive care unit. 2007:135-143

[11] Fowler RA, Sabur N, Li P, Juurlink DN, Pinto R, Hladunewich MA, et al. Sex- and age-based differences in the delivery and outcomes of critical care. Canadian Medical Association Journal (CMAJ). 2009;**177**(12):1513-1519

[12] Olaya B, Domènech-abella J, Victoria M, Lara E, Félix F, Rico-uribe LA, et al. All-cause mortality and multimorbidity in older adults: The role of social support and loneliness. Experimental Gerontology [Internet]. 2017;**99**(March):120-126. DOI: 10.1016/j.exger.2017.10.001

[13] Hanlon P, Nicholl BI, Jani BD, Lee D, Mcqueenie R, Mair FS. Articles frailty and pre-frailty in middle-aged and older adults and its association with multimorbidity and mortality: A prospective analysis of 493 737 UK Biobank participants. The Lancet Public Health [Internet];**3**(7):e323-e332. DOI: 10.1016/S2468-2667(18)30091-4

[14] Vosylius S, Sipylaite J, Ivaskevicius J. Determinants of outcome in elderly patients admitted to the intensive care unit. Age Ageing. 2005;**34**(2):157-162

[15] Ghavarskhar F, Matlabi H, Gharibi F, Sertyesilisik B. Architecture | review article. A systematic review to compare residential care facilities for older people in developed countries: Practical implementations for Iran. Cogent Social Sciences [Internet]. 2018;**4**:1-21. DOI: 10.1080/23311886.2018.1478493

[16] Stein FDC. Prognostic factors in elderly patients admitted in the intensive care unit. 2009;**21**(1):255-261

www.ingramcontent.com/pod-product-compliance
Lightning Source LLC
Chambersburg PA
CBHW081240190326
41458CB00016B/5854